BRYAN APPLEYARD was born in Manchester and was educated at Bolton School and King's College, Cambridge. He is currently a special feature writer for the *Sunday Times*. He has also written for *The Times*, the *Daily Telegraph*, the *New York Times* and *Vanity Fair*, among others, and has three times been named Feature Writer of the Year and twice commended at the British Press Awards. He is the author of several previous books, the most recent of which is *Aliens: Why They Are Here*, also published by Simon & Schuster. He lives in London.

For more information visit www.bryanappleyard.com

HOW TO LIVE FOREVER OR DIE TRYING

On the New Immortality

BRYAN APPLEYARD

SIMON &
SCHUSTER

London · New York · Sydney · Toronto

A CBS COMPANY

First published in Great Britain by Simon & Schuster UK Ltd, 2007
A CBS COMPANY

1 3 5 7 9 10 8 6 4 2

Simon & Schuster UK Ltd
Africa House
64–78 Kingsway
London WC2B 6AH

www.simonsays.co.uk

Simon & Schuster Australia
Sydney

A CIP catalogue record for this book
is available from the British Library.

ISBN-13: 978-0-7432-6868-4
ISBN-10: 0-7432-6868-7

Printed and bound in Great Britain by
CPI Bath

For Christena

Contents

Acknowledgements

Numerous people have spoken to me informally on the subject of immortality, but I would particularly like to thank the following for granting me more formal interviews: James Ballard, John Bond, Nick Bostrom, Stephen Braude, Benjamin Colby, Damaso Crespo, Kate Davidson, Gregory Fahy, David Gobel, Aubrey de Grey, John Harris, Russell Hepple, Steve Horrobin, James Hughes, Tanya Jones, Tom Kirkwood, Bruce Klein, James Larrick, Max More, Michael Rose, Roger Scruton, Rafal Smigrodzki, Joe Waynick, Michael West, Eliezer Yudkowsky.

By my troth, I care not; a man can die but once; we owe God a death.

William Shakespeare

Introduction:

Cancelling the Debt

The Debt

This book is inspired by the possibility of human life extension. Developments in a number of scientific disciplines suggest that we may soon be able to increase life expectancies from the seventy- to eighty-year range now seen in the richest countries to well over a hundred and, perhaps, to over a thousand. We shall, in one sense, have made ourselves immortal. We shall not be immortal in the sense that we cannot die; plainly we could still be killed in a car accident or by a cosmic event such as an asteroid striking the earth. But we could not be killed by disease or age, our bodies would be immune to infection, dysfunction or the ravages of time. We would be medically immortal.

Some say this will happen quickly – within, perhaps, thirty years with the first clear signs that we are on the right track appearing within the next decade. Others think we are at least a century or two away from attaining medical immortality. Some consider it completely unattainable. But the majority of scientists and thinkers in this area now consider life extension and even medical immortality possible and likely. Not long ago, most would have said it was out of the question, that death at or well before the absolute maximum age of something like 122 was inevitable. (That was the age at which Jean Louise Calment died on 4 August 1977. She has the most credible claim to be the longest-lived human ever, almost all other claims having been discredited. Maria Olivia da Silva, a Brazilian, is said to have been born in February 1880, but, so far, this has not been verified.)

The basis of this shift from unattainable to feasible is not generally understood. It involves a transformation in our conception of human biology and an expansion of our capacity to intervene in its workings that may yet prove to be at least as momentous as the discoveries of Copernicus, Galileo, Newton, Darwin or Einstein. I shall explain this scientific transformation in some detail in Chapter Two.

But Copernicus to Einstein is not the only tradition that is at issue here. There are also the traditions that run from Buddha to Mohammed and from Plato to Wittgenstein, the traditions of religion and philosophy. Our relatively brief lives and our routine proximity to the deaths of ourselves and others are the foundations of everything we have ever thought or believed. Neither religion nor philosophy necessarily promises immortality, but each offers ways of coming to terms with or giving meaning to death and, therefore, life. If death is to be postponed indefinitely, then both religion and philosophy face fundamental crises.

Of course, many other traditions – of politics, art, commerce and culture – are also at stake. In truth, it is difficult to think of any aspect of human life that would not face similar crises. What, for example, would be the meaning of the greatest works of the human imagination to a medical immortal? Shakespeare's sonnets may be said to be about the brevity of life and the painful transience of human love and beauty. But if we lived for a thousand years or more in a condition of youthful health and vitality – the postulated life-extension technologies promise to hold us permanently in our late twenties – then would we come to see these poems as the curious remnants of an antique world rather than urgent expressions of the deepest truths of our predicament? Would any art of the past survive this revolution with its dignity intact? Would there be any art of the future?

Many may think that, as they suffer from no illusions, fantasies or sensitivities, new life-extension technologies are nothing but good news, simple additions to the portfolio of benefits delivered by modern technology. But their worlds are also threatened. For example, the language of relationships is the vernacular of our contemporary, secular life. What would our precious relationships look like to medical immortals? Love itself would have to be redefined. Romantic love depends for its very meaning on the promise that it will last forever. But 'forever' now means no more than, say, fifty years, the average span, in other words, of the human life from falling in love to death. If falling in love actually meant a commitment for a thousand or more years, then 'forever' starts to take on a new meaning. Love is suddenly relativised, its significance thrown into doubt.

There remains, of course, love of self and surely in that context life extension must be an unalloyed good. Life extension must mean extension of the self and the cultivation of the self is, alongside relationships, the supreme contemporary preoccupation. But even here there are problems. How much cultivation of the self can we take? There will only ever be so many gadgets to buy, so many days we can spend at the gym or beauty parlour – though these may well be unnecessary activities in the new world order – so much sex we can have, so many cars we can drive. Perhaps medically immortal selves will seek alternative spiritual or intellectual diversions as the wealthier mortal selves, disillusioned with getting and spending, already do in increasing numbers. Maybe these will see us through the long centuries of life. Or maybe none of these things will matter as we shall not be just one self in the future but many. The human brain already struggles to cope with the memories of eighty years, what would it do with those of more than a thousand years? The average fifty-year-old can only fleetingly put himself in the mind and imagination of his ten-year-old self, would a five-hundred-year-old even be able to see it as the same self? Perhaps medical immortals will simply have to resign themselves to amnesia, to becoming serial, forgetful selves.

Would medical immortals go to war? Would they form nations? Would they be democrats? Would they go shopping? Would they destroy the environment? The promise of extreme longevity is, according to your temperament, either a threat or a wish that nothing whatsoever will remain the same.

It is the supreme challenge of science. Arguments about the impact of science and technology upon ways of life are tediously familiar. To the church, Galileo threatened orthodoxy; to the romantics, the Industrial Revolution threatened the rural paradise and the authenticity of craft; to the religious, Darwinism threatened the faith; to the pacifist, nuclear power offered only more terrible wars; to the environmentalist, economic growth threatened global destruction; to the conservative, bio-technological enhancement threatened a destruction of human nature. But life extension to the point of medical immortality condenses all these conflicts into a single issue. All the ambivalence we feel about scientific progress is condensed in the question: do we want much longer lives?

One can only speak for oneself and, in this book, that is

exactly what I do. This is about what I feel (and, autobio-
graphically, why I feel it) about medical immortality, about
my responses to the arguments of the immortalists or pro-
longevists and the deathists, bio-conservatives or just plain
Luddites. On the offer of immortality itself, I began this project as a confirmed deathist. Death, I was sure, gave meaning
to life, at least the only meaning we could imagine. Like
Wittgenstein, I would wonder to what puzzle immortality
was the solution. Subsequently, I found that my curiosity
began to get the better of this philosophically pure position.
Lying on my deathbed, would I refuse the treatment that
would take me back to my late twenties and perfect health?
This, surely, is the one offer nobody could refuse.

Because I am considering the culture and history of immortality, the actual science of life extension is but one of my
concerns. There are a number of books listed in the bibli-
ography that tell the scientific story more fully. For my
purposes, a number of broad scientific concepts and certain
key personalities are all that is necessary. They underpin but
they do not wholly define my theme. Also I am not attempting – because I am not qualified – to assess the science. I do
not know whether immortality is imminent, in the distant
future or wholly impossible. All I know is that many people
think it is imminent and current scientific evidence suggests it
may be. Even if human life extension turns out to be a fantasy, the possibility is now in the air and is already
conditioning our imaginations.

What I am presenting here is more of an anthology or a
meditation than an argument. It is an anthology of experience, events, memories, arguments and evocations and a
meditation on what my/our life ultimately is. And also the
stories of the frequently strange and driven people who have
become involved in the debates and practicalities of life
extension. The issue may be seen as simple when posed as

the, for the moment, hypothetical question: would you accept this treatment? But, when seen in the round, it becomes complex but also revealing.

In this context, I should also say that, though personal, this book is not only concerned with my opinions. Many views are expressed in this book; I shall do my best to make it clear when they are mine. For the moment, it is best to assume I have no opinions whatsoever on the subjects discussed. This is almost true.

Ultimately, the pursuit of life extension or medical immortality is a continuation of the ancient pursuit of the conquest of death, either by giving it meaning or by survival in this life or some other. It is the scientific version of the oldest human aspiration, which is either to evade oblivion or to embrace it with the consolatory knowledge that one's life has acquired significance. Shakespeare, as usual, found the single exact word to capture what is at stake here. The word is 'owe'. Feeble in *Henry V* says 'we owe God a death'. For Feeble, to be born is to be indebted. Our death settles the account. This feels like a profoundly true statement. I shall now try to work out why it is. Or why it isn't.

The Pay-Off

In recent years, a fundamental shift has taken place in our attitudes to the ageing process and to the possibility that human life can be extended, perhaps indefinitely. This is what historians of science call a 'paradigm shift', a basic change of perspective comparable to the revolution in physics brought about by relativity and quantum theory in the early twentieth century or, more appropriately, to the transformation of biology that followed the publication of Charles Darwin's *On the Origin of Species* in 1859. This shift has not yet penetrated the lay imagination. The contemporary boosters for immortality are, as a young anthropologist from New York observed to me, pioneers, the advance guard of a revolution which will, if they are right, change human history. Indeed, it will change that history into something post-human, into a new and, so they claim, 'higher' order of consciousness. The immortal beings a thousand years hence will look back at us with uncomprehending pity. How could we endure the misery of such brief lives and the chaos and confusion of our unre-formed animal natures?

If the immortalists are right, this transformation of the human has already begun. There is now a significant industry consisting of many brilliant and often evangelical individuals, all of them driven by the conviction that the human body can be improved, perhaps perfected. The rapid growth of biolog-ical knowledge since the decoding of DNA in 1953 as well as fundamental conceptual changes about the way we view the human body has led us to a new perspective on our lives and deaths. Ideas are now in the air which promise or threaten to increase human life expectancy significantly.

Is there any limit to this process? The most ardent advo-cates of life extension say there is not. The body is a machine like any other, they claim, and can be fixed. In the next few decades, we can reasonably expect to extend life expectancies to 150 or beyond. People will be then living long enough to benefit from yet more advances in medical technology that will extend their lives still further. Ultimately, the forward movement of technology will outstrip our own forward movement through time, and death, the old enemy, will have been vanquished. As a result of this 'escape velocity' effect, the first human to live a thousand years, it has been said, may have already been born.

(There is one ingenious calculation of how long such a person would live. The gerontologist Steven Austad studied death rates among children of about eleven, the age at which people are least likely to die since they have survived the perils of childhood and have yet to suffer the deteriorations of age. They are rather like medical immortals in that they are most likely to die as a result of an accident. The death rates of eleven-year-olds should, therefore, be comparable to those of immortals. Using death rates in eleven-year-olds, Austad calculated that a medical immortal would have a life expectancy of 1200 years. Austad has also bet $500 million that somebody living in 2001 will still be alive and sentient in 2150; it is a wager he says he is 'feeling very good about'.)

This is what has fired the imaginations and enthusiasm of the immortalists. If, they say, such momentous developments really are imminent, then we must get on with not just anti-ageing but also anti-death research as quickly as possible. Medical research aims at merely stalling the dying process, it must be about conquering death. Lives are at stake. This is not simply a scientific project, it is a cause, the justice and urgency of which is made evident daily by our own wrinkling skins and aching joints as well as by the death throes of our loved ones.

There is also a slightly less noble, more specifically contemporary impulse behind all this. The possibility that we are within reach of these technologies has placed a set of those alive today in a tricky and frustrating position. This is the baby boomer set, those born in the years after the Second World War. I find myself a member of this materially fortunate but spiritually troubled cohort. In the West, especially in the United States, these people – something stops me saying 'we' – have enjoyed health and prosperity unprecedented in human history. But now, aged between, say, forty-five and sixty, they are facing decrepitude. In the sixties, they sang along with The Who – 'I hope I die before I get old' – but those that survived now find this hope dashed.

'As baby boomers age and their parents die,' observe

Colleen McDannell and Bernhard Lang in their book *Heaven: A History*, 'death has become a hot topic. In Europe, and perhaps even more in the United States, there is now a consumer market for products that speak to our fantasies about life after death.'

Boomers confront old age and the prospect of the freedoms and luxuries they have enjoyed being snatched from them as death, the great leveller, consigns them to rot in the same earth as less fortunate generations. Yet now, they are told, we may be within two or three decades of the technology that will postpone and may ultimately save them from this fate. So many things have been fixed in the post-war era, from polio to computer crashes, why not also death?

But, for the baby boomers, the window of opportunity is both tantalisingly close and frighteningly distant. 'A small minority of older boomers', tease Ray Kurzweil and Terry Grossman, boomers both, in their book *Fantastic Voyage: Live Long Enough to Live For Ever*, 'will make it past this impending critical threshold. You can be among them.'

It is hard not to feel the pressure of such offers, hard not to find oneself considering the purchase of countless dietary supplements and a blood pressure machine. What else is on offer? Only oblivion. Baby boomers have always loved exclusive clubs, this is the most exclusive club of all, a club of immortal post-humans, a club of gods.

But, if we can achieve life extension in humans within thirty years, then the boomers will have to wait until they are between seventy-five and ninety. They will have first to survive and, secondly, maintain a reasonable degree of bodily health as the technologies may not work on the decrepit. To die a year or a day before the membership lists open, to be among the last to die 'young', would be intolerable.

'That', as one boomer scientist put it to me, 'would suck.'

Since the seventies, wealthy boomers have tended to be

fussy about their health, exercising, dieting and taking supplements. But those who know about the possibility of life
extension have gone much further. I have encountered self-
prescribing doctors using drugs to keep their blood pressures
and cholesterol levels at phenomenally low levels, scientists
taking up to 250 supplements a day and exercising furiously
and, most extreme of all, calorie restrictionists living on only
two thirds of the food intake once thought necessary. Not
much of a life, you may say, but, on the other hand, if it
works as planned then one day they will be able to abandon
all these punishing regimes and live it up as they did in the
sixties.

Meanwhile, in Scottsdale, Arizona, I saw the huge
Dewars – stainless steel Thermos flasks – in which heads and
whole bodies are kept deep frozen. These are the people who
have been frozen on death in the hope that future technology
will thaw them out and fix whatever it was that killed them.
This is, perhaps, the most literal way of leaping the temporal
gap between now and the biologically more adept future.

Eternity is on offer. Well, perhaps not quite, as Austad
makes clear. The medically fixed body will still be a physical,
destroyable presence in the world. Yet perhaps Austad is
overly pessimistic because, with the prospect of effective
immortality before them, people might go to greater lengths
to avoid fatal accidents. They will have more to lose. He may
also be pessimistic because he underestimates just how far the
technology can go.

Nanotechnology – engineering at the level of the nanometre or one millionth of a millimetre – could either make
our bodies more accident-proof or it could reconstruct them.
Taken to hospital after a car crash, you would have billions of
tiny machines injected into your bloodstream to repair the
damage.

On the other hand, 1200 years may be optimistic because

it is just too long. We might grow bored. Friendships, marriages and love might die. Children might come to seem a futile consolation. Memories and feeling would fade. Perhaps, long before the accident, we would choose to pay God back.

The Price

So would immortality – either medical or actual – be a good or a bad thing? The question is worth asking now not just because of the technology, but also for three other reasons.

The very fact that the possibility is seriously being considered tells us something about the age in which we live and its aspirations, its ideas, in fact, of heaven.

Secondly, the desire for some kind of immortality has been a consistent feature of every human society. Our version of that desire is but the latest episode in a long and distinguished but admittedly bloody history.

Thirdly, death is the issue and that is a particular problem for secular, materially successful societies. As two very percipient writers on the subject – Philippe Aries and Geoffrey Gorer – have shown, our contemporary way of dealing with death is the least adequate in human history. We have invented a new way of dying, surrounded by strangers in hospitals and nursing homes, and fear any reminder of death and decay.

'They clearly no longer had any guidance from ritual,' wrote Gorer of his embarrassed friends who turned away from his expressions of grief at the death of his brother, 'as to the way to treat a self-confessed mourner . . .'

That was in 1965. Today Gorer might have noted how we distance decay even more brutally by mocking the old, the only group that can now be openly and cruelly abused. The jokes seen daily on television at the expense of the old could not be made at the expense of blacks, Jews or Muslims. But we are not afraid of the old in the same way we are of those other groups. We don't fear their wrath, we fear their condition – their smell, their wrinkled skin and their sexually undesirable bodies – and so we laugh because admitting to our fears would be counter-therapeutic.

In a way, the pursuit of medical immortality is just a further extension of this strategy of evasion. Aries ends *The Hour of Our Death*, his great history of death, by defining two distinctive modern attitudes. The first is denial, the second is that of 'a small elite of anthropologists, psychologists, and sociologists' who wish to 'humanise' death: 'Death must simply become the discreet but dignified exit of a peaceful person from a helpful society that is not torn, not even overly upset by the idea of a biological transition without significance, without pain or suffering and ultimately without fear.'

Aries dreamt of secular rituals for a secular Utopia. Fair enough. But, surely, a far more bracingly secular dream is to render all such rituals unnecessary, to banish death, to join the charge of the immortalists against the old foe. This is the third modern attitude that has emerged since Aries published his book in 1977 – to deny death not by averting our gaze but by finding the cure.

But what would be the price of that cure, the cost of buying ourselves out of the debt to God? Is it worth paying? It is easy to say no, that it is good that people die to make way for new generations, the love of our own children gives transcendent virtue to such a sentiment. But if, on your deathbed, the offer was seriously made, how would you respond? Perhaps you would say you did not wish to live on old and decrepit. But, if this new technology works, that will not happen, you will be rejuvenated, returned, ideally, to the condition you were in in your late twenties and you would be maintained at that age until killed by an accident or by your own hand or forever. Why not, therefore, take the pill?

After all, as Michael West of Advanced Cell Technologies put it to me, 'We can always die, it's easy to die.' Shakespeare's Juliet said much the same: 'If all else fail, myself have power to die.'

But to understand the full significance of this offer of medical immortality, it is necessary to go back to the basics of the human condition. Every human that has ever lived has lived with the knowledge: I must die. Not just dying but also knowing we must is the defining characteristic of the species. Humans – *Homo sapiens* – are animals that know and the thing they know with the most certainty, dread and incredulity is that they must die.

Ancient Greeks called humans 'mortals', partly to distinguish them from immortal gods, but also to distinguish them from the whole of the rest of creation. Animals and plants were thought not to die because they were not individuals. And, beyond the earth, the cosmos persisted in timeless, changeless stasis. All of nature was immortal. Man alone rose up, decayed and died. He was not just a mortal, he was *the* mortal. 'Man', wrote W.B. Yeats, 'has created death.' And Jorge Luis Borges wrote, 'To be immortal is commonplace; except for man, all creatures are immortal, for they are ignorant of death . . .'

Later generations may have shed those views of animals and the cosmos, but the central human predicament – that we must die and know about it – remained. Religions sometimes promised a life *beyond* death and, occasionally, some suggested that not dying at all was a possibility. But, on the whole, humans, once past childhood, have always lived with the certain knowledge that they must die. They acquire this knowledge because of the spectacle of others not merely dying but also growing old. Nothing can be more certain than death; with every passing year, our bodies provide the evidence.

Human civilisation is a response to this knowledge. The moment the ape became introspective, he began to ponder his own extinction with rank incredulity. Some graves of Neanderthals were decorated with flowers, and Palaeolithic burial mounds were far more enduring than the homes of the living. We do not know exactly what such things meant, but we do know they meant that there was no possibility of mere blank acceptance of extinction. Later, of course, the marks became less ambiguous. Every temple, shrine, church, monument and memorial testified to a conviction that death was not a complete cessation. Even if the individual was lost, the civilisation continued. Indeed, there has probably never been a book written, music composed or picture painted that does not concern the matter of death and the possibility of some kind of immortality. No human society has ever been indifferent to death and none has ever been able to accept with any kind of equanimity the apparently obvious meaning of the word: the total extinction of the individual.

Self-consciousness thus seems to be a trap. It makes a world that seems external to itself. Yet that world, the world as seen by the seer, is destined to vanish utterly. We cannot even console ourselves with the thought that it continues for others because the world I see is the world defined by my self-consciousness alone. It dies with me. The idea is beyond belief.

This incredulity even survives the sight of the death of others. As Tolstoy observed in *The Death of Ivan Ilyich*, '. . . the mere fact of the death of an intimate associate aroused, as is usual, in all who heard of it, a complacent feeling that "it is he who is dead, and not I"'. And Thomas à Kempis in *The Imitation of Christ* advises good Christians, 'If you have ever seen anyone die, remember that you, too, must travel the same road.' What is extraordinary is the fact that the complacency is real and the advice is necessary when death is so obviously all around us. We need these constant reminders because our incredulity at the possibility of our own death makes our capacity for denial limitless.

But denial is not just a matter of egotism, blind faith or the inability to face reality, it is logically consistent.

'My death is not an event in the knowable world of objects,' writes Zygmunt Bauman, echoing both Ludwig Wittgenstein's remark that death is not an event in life and François de La Rochefoucauld's, 'One cannot look directly at either the sun or death.' Also Sigmund Freud observed that, fundamentally, no man believes in his own death. It is not a thing in his world.

An absolute impossibility dominates our lives – the replacement of this something by nothing. What could nothing possibly be? In fact, nothing, the abyss, is really only a concept of the modern era. Until recently, our incredulity succeeded in defeating our reason and insisted on establishing something that was not nothing. Nothing did not exist in the past; there was, instead, the vast panoply of meanings and monuments.

Spanish-American philosopher George Santayana made the point more elegantly:

Confidence in living forever is anterior to the discovery that all men are mortal and to the discovery that the thinker himself is a man. These discoveries flatly contradict that confidence, in the form in which it originally presents itself, and all doctrines of immortality which adult philosophy can entertain are more or less subterfuges and after-thoughts by which the observed fact of mortality and the native inconceivability of death are more or less clumsily reconciled.

Everybody dies, therefore I must die. This being inconceivable, we invent immortality and these inventions are civilisation.

But science threatened these inventions by describing a physical universe that not only had no need of God but also had no need of us. We flickered into and out of existence with the same empty brevity as a shooting star. Science drew our attention to what seemed to be the undeniable facts of the case.

'You're born, it's a great ride and you die. That's it,' as James Larrick, doctor and micro-biological entrepreneur, put it to me. Or, more accurately for most people, life is hard, then you die. Now, however, science is saying these may not be the facts of the case. Death may no longer be the one clear fact of life. It can be postponed indefinitely, maybe even abolished. What happens then to people who have defined themselves by death?

Probably they cease to be human. Some, like Francis Fukuyama and Leon Kass, are appalled by the prospect of abandoning our humanity. Others, like the thinkers in the World Transhumanist Association, welcome the idea. What, they ask, is so great about being human, being driven mad by dreams made impossible by the dying animal to which we are tethered? Nature, as Ray Kurzweil observes, is 'dramatically suboptimal' so why not just fix the human condition? It is hard to argue when our paradoxical civilisation is built not just upon death but also upon the sustenance of life.

'All the scriptures are pretty clear,' said Aubrey de Grey, one of the leading scientists in this area, 'hastening death is deprecated and, if something is killing people, we are more or less instructed to do something about it.'

'In any consistent program of meliorism,' wrote immortality historian Gerald Gruman, 'the prolongation of life must have a significant place . . .'

To the meliorists I have met, the word 'significant' does not do justice to their commitment to the simple cause of not dying. In their eyes, the prolongation of life has become the *only* serious project for our species. The immortalists are looking for the big pay-off, not the settling of the account with God, but the revelation that we owe him nothing and we never did. All deals are off.

That we now face a rapid and fundamental transformation of the world through science and technology, I do not doubt. This transformation may be unambiguously catastrophic, involving either environmental collapse or the destruction of our civilisation through the use of our advanced weaponry. Or it may be ambiguous, involving technologies of human life extension and/or transformation through biology or computer science. Either way, something has started to happen, something that may be very like what I attempt to describe in this book.

But now it is time to go to the Deep South and join the immortalists at the Immortality Institute.

1

The Atlanta Braves

Bruce Klein founded The Immortality Institute (Imminst) in 2002 as a non-profit organisation with the aim of 'conquering the blight of involuntary death'. Klein was brought up in the town of Americus, 'a jewel of Georgia', in Bible Belt America, the deep south. 'Yeah, I'm a southern redneck!' he jokes. His family was not especially religious, though he did observe the Catholicism of his mother until the age of eleven when he took a phone call from their priest.

'I said to him I didn't believe any more. He got kind of upset and I hung up the phone. It was some kind of visceral thing.'

Klein was thirty-one when I met him at Imminst's conference at the Georgia Tech Conference Center, Atlanta, in November 2005. The conference turned out to be a snapshot of the immortalist front line. It is a movement that is part cult and part serious science. But all were united by the fervency of their belief in the rightness of the project of extending life and by their vehement rejection of deathism and scepticism. The participants saw themselves as visionaries and frequently beleaguered pioneers of the only new frontier left to mankind.

Klein is a groomed, fit-looking man. His wife and 'wonderful friend', Susan Fonseca-Klein, co-founder and director of the institute, is round-faced and pretty. Together, they have the air not of a threateningly glamorous but of a consolingly ideal couple – young, healthy, good-natured, extravagantly friendly, ambitious, optimistic, glowing. One could imagine them in an advertisement for breakfast cereal.

Most of their work is involved with running Imminst, though Klein does say he manages some property and investments. His degree from the University of Georgia is in finance. He had just moved from Atlanta to Bethesda, Maryland. He is also president of Bethesda-based Novamente, a small firm devoted to the construction and commercialisation of the Novamente AI Engine, an 'artifical general intelligence oriented software system', and he wished to be closer to that project and its presiding thinker Ben Goertzel.

Goertzel, who was also at the conference, is aggressively scruffy with tangled, heavy metal hair and jeans barely clinging to his hips. As he queued to ask a question of one of the speakers, I took him for a bum who had wandered in off the empty downtown streets and was preparing myself for an embarrassing incident culminating in his ejection from the hall. In fact, he was himself a speaker and a maths professor, though whatever normality that implies is swiftly detonated by the discovery that his first son is named Zarathustra Amadeus and his second Zebulon Ulysses. The more restrained Klein is, in spite of his wife's protests, putting off having children until he has made the world 'a safer place', ideally by banishing death.

Along with increasing numbers of people in the immortality field, Klein believes artificial intelligence may be the best way forward, hence his new partnership with Goertzel. There are two possibilities arising from AI. Either a super-intelligent computer could master the medical problems of human ageing that currently baffle us or, more speculatively, we could back-up our personalities by downloading them on to such a machine.

Imminst has been highly successful. It is primarily web-based – you can find it at www.imminst.org – and the quality and responsiveness of its site is extremely high. The moment I joined, some months before the conference, I was (electronically) welcomed by Klein and invited to host a web chat, which I did rather sleepily between one and two in the morning. Atlanta is five hours behind my house in Stiffkey, Norfolk.

Within the context of the pursuit of immortality, Imminst fills a gap in a very crowded field. Alcor in Scottsdale, Arizona, and the Cryonics Institute in Clinton, Michigan, specialise in advocating and practising the deep freezing of people immediately after death in the hope that they can be revived by superior medical technology at some point in the future. The Extropy Institute and the World Transhumanist Association focus on all the ways in which we can technologically transcend our biological condition. In Silicon Valley, California, the Singularity Institute for Artificial Intelligence pursues the AI route, particularly studying the ways in which we could guarantee the 'friendliness' of any such machine. SENS (Strategies for Engineered Negligible Senescence) follows a tightly focused medical programme defined by Aubrey de Grey, a scientist based in Cambridge in the UK. The American Academy of Anti-Aging Medicine seeks to push the boundaries of mainstream medicine in the direction of increased longevity. The Methuselah Foundation primarily runs the Mprize aimed at encouraging research into increasing longevity in mice. And so on. But only Imminst acts as an open-minded forum for all ideas about increasing human longevity. It is neither general like Extropy nor specific like Alcor, SENS or the Singularity Institute, it is simply concerned with the pursuit of human immortality by whatever means seem most promising.

Why? Because, says Klein, 'oblivion is the issue'.

He says: 'I came to a point about five years ago where I realised I can't do all of this unless I'm alive . . . The thing that human beings, I think, are evolved to do is put the issue of oblivion to one side. What I try to do is address that problem with writings, with film scripts and the thing is not only to address it but to provide a solution, the solution of infinite life span.'

He speaks, as does everybody in this business, of the 150,000 people who die in the world every day, 100,000 of them from the diseases of old age. For him, this is not acceptably explained as the natural order of things, rather it is a disaster to which we are called to respond.

'I call it the Silent Tsunami, every day more than 100,000 people die quietly and acceptingly, saying their time has come or some other euphemism. But, with a real tsunami, they say this is a tragedy, we must do things to prevent this in the future.'

Most people who have become immortalists do so because of this paradox. We are horrified by the millions of deaths caused by wars or natural disasters. Humanely, we are determined, in the present, to help and, in the future, to do what we can to prevent such things happening again. But, on the other hand, confronted by this other daily carnage, this background slaughter, we pass by on the other side, uncaring, almost unnoticing except when we or those we know are involved.

Perhaps we do so because we know we all must die. But that, say the immortalists, is no longer true or need not be in the near future. Science has now advanced to the point where we can begin to imagine solutions. Indeed, our science has progressed so far that we are *morally bound* to seek solutions, just as we would be morally bound to prevent a real tsunami if we knew how. Some further assert that the Western tradition requires that absolute value be accorded to every individual life. And it is that very Western tradition, as expressed through the scientific method, that is now offering us the opportunity to banish death.

Such arguments provoke opposition from what the immortalists call 'deathists', those who have attacked the pursuit of immortality as wrong-headed, futile or even dangerous in that it threatens to destroy our human nature, the evolved basis of our moral perspective. Even the Vatican has stepped in to attack the transhumanist movement. The immortalists, like all such groupings, derive yet more energy and conviction from these external assaults.

So, back at Atlanta, the immortalists were inspired to find they were facing two further attacks from much closer to home which were to set the conference alight.

Aubrey de Grey is, perhaps, the most astonishing figure in the entire immortality movement. He seems to have sprung from the pages of a Dostoyevsky novel, a saint or a demon but certainly nothing in between. He has a huge beard and whiskers and hair as long as but straighter than Goertzel's which he ties back in a ponytail with a scrunchy. His face is pale and often drawn. It is that of a driven or even possessed man. It is also somewhat ageless though he is, in fact, in his early forties. He dresses in denim and sneakers and speaks with immense assurance in perfect sentences and paragraphs. His voice is high and penetrating. I had not allowed for his extreme visual and auditory impact when I met him at the Groucho Club in London. For two hours he sat on the edge of a sofa and reduced the London media crowd to stunned silence as he described to me his 'engineering' strategy to defeat ageing. At Atlanta, he is hailed by the immortalists as if he were a rock star. After the conference, he drinks beer – he *loves* beer – in the bar and held court until the early hours of the morning. I had seen him do exactly the same at his own SENS conference a few months earlier. De Grey's manner is startling but attractive. Even his enemies admit he is an immensely likeable man.

His enemies also admit that he is brilliant. But he is a maverick, a figure not strictly welcome at the medical and biological high table. He is, for a start, self taught. His original discipline was computer science and the one actual job he has at Cambridge is as a computer scientist in the Department of Genetics. He became interested in biology when he married the geneticist Adelaide Carpenter, who is nineteen years older than him, in 1991. He has since self-educated his way to a PhD and to global prominence as the leader of the immortalists. He actually hates the word 'immortal' as he merely aims to conquer ageing and rejuvenate people in such a way that they will cease to age.

He also creates enemies by his insistence that the problem of ageing cannot be solved by pure science, but by engineering. Scientists try to learn everything they can about a problem; engineers limit their research to what they *need* to know to fix it. Thus, for example, a scientist may spend a lifetime investigating the metabolic debris that accumulates in the ageing human cell; an engineer would simply work out ways of removing the debris and restoring the cell's function. Why and how it accumulated in the first place are not his concern. Scientists, not surprisingly, note with some rancour the implied suggestion that much of their lives are wasted on the futile pursuit of total wisdom.

De Grey is also a publicist. He attracts and revels in press coverage, generating headlines around the world by claiming that life extension, perhaps even medical immortality, may be possible within thirty years. He does this for the perfectly valid reason that he believes publicity will bring funding to anti-ageing research. But such publicity seeking makes enemies of those more used to a lower profile and more cautious in the politics of research grants. I know de Grey has been asked to remove links to a more mainstream website from his own SENS site and he has done so. Some feel tainted by association.

But, just before the Atlanta conference, polite disdain for his style, his methods and his manner had exploded into something quite different. De Grey had been the cover story of the February 2005 issue of *Technology Review*, the 'magazine of innovation' of the Massachusetts Institute of Technology. Sherwin Nuland had profiled de Grey. Nuland is an important figure in my story and I shall return to him in another context. He is a very distinguished doctor – professor of surgery at Yale's School of Medicine – and an exceptional writer, author of the formidable *How We Die*, a book that forces us to confront the usually appalling physical reality of dying but also, crucially, argues for an acceptance of that reality. Nuland was, in short, predisposed to disagree with de Grey's entire project because, like Kass, like Fukuyama, he believes that death is a good thing for our species.

The article is, indeed, an elegant hatchet job, suggesting that many of de Grey's theoretical solutions may be 'little more than slogans'. Philosophically, Nuland questions 'the ultimate leap of ingenious argument that would do a sophist proud' whereby immortalists suggest that by not pursuing life extension, we are hastening death. Most seriously of all, he suggests de Grey is a threat to the world – 'the most likable eccentrics are sometimes the most dangerous'.

'With the passion of a single-minded zealot crusading against time,' Nuland wrote, 'he has issued the ultimate challenge, I believe, to our entire concept of the meaning of humanness. Paradoxically, his clarion call to action is the message neither of a madman nor a bad man, but of a brilliant, beneficent man of goodwill, who wants only for civilization to fulfil the highest hopes ... It is a good thing that his grand design will almost certainly not succeed. Were it otherwise, he would surely destroy us in attempting to preserve us.'

In his editorial, the magazine's editor, Jason Pontin, used Nuland's article as the basis for a crude, personal attack on de Grey:

> But what struck me is that he is a troll. For all de Grey's vaulting ambitions, what Sherwin Nuland saw from the outside was pathetically circumscribed. In his waking life, de Grey ... dresses like a shabby graduate student and affects Rip Van Winkle's beard; he has no children; he has few interests outside the science of biogerontology; he drinks too much beer. Although he is only forty-one, the signs of decay are strongly marked on his face. His ideas are trollish, too. ... Immortality might be okay for de Grey, but an entire world of the same superagenarians thinking the same kinds of thoughts forever would be terrible.

Pontin drove the point home by saying on his contents page that Nuland found de Grey 'brilliant – but also nuts'. This is not true, Nuland did not find that, and neither is it true that de Grey drinks too much beer. He may love beer, he may make a fuss about beer, but I've only ever seen him drink it in, by my standards, moderation.

Worse was to come. In the November 2005 issue of *EMBO Reports*, the journal of the European Molecular Biology Organization, twenty-eight leading scientists, including Tom

Kirkwood, S. Jay Olshansky and Richard A. Miller, signed a three-page Viewpoint piece attacking de Grey and the whole SENS agenda. His scheme, they said, was a farrago, a programme that 'falls into the realms of fantasy' and which depended on the cooperation of gullible journalists. De Grey was threatening to distort research priorities through 'clever marketing' that was 'a poor substitute for scientific thought'. They argue that de Grey's intervention comes at a difficult moment for ageing research, 'a discipline that is only just emerging from a reputation for charlatanry'. Wild claims will only damage the gradual ascent of the discipline into full respectability.

'De Grey's credibility, among those who do not know his ideas well enough to understand their weaknesses, lies partly in his claims that his ideas have been judged interesting and provocative by mainstream gerontologists. The authors of this article, proud of our roles as representative mainstream biogerontologists, wish to dissociate ourselves from the cadre of those impressed by de Grey's ideas in their present state.'

EMBO Reports did not, like *Technology Review*, endorse the article in an editorial, but rather took, in the event, the more entertaining option of giving de Grey a right of reply in the same issue. He delights in his powers of sarcasm. And, so of the angry scientists' assertion that none of his ideas have ever been shown to extend the life of any organism *in isolation*, he says: 'I do not recall Henry Ford alerting potential customers that the components of a car – in isolation – remain obstinately stationary when burning petrol is poured on them, nor do I recall his being castigated for this omission.'

He concludes:

They do not challenge my arguments that adherence to biologically and politically naive rhetoric is precisely why gerontology continues to have such trouble impressing policy makers, yet they steadfastly defend that rhetoric as if somehow one more push will change everything. I offer no apology for using media interest in life extension to make the biology of ageing an exception to Planck's observation that science advances funeral by funeral: lives, lots of them, are at stake.

De Grey, welcomed to the Atlanta stage with whoops of approval, made these same points in his speech and brought the house down. De Grey may be English but he has a natural affinity with what David Nye, a British academic, has called, 'the American technological sublime'. Immortalists one, we felt, deathists nil.

The battlefield, by the time of the conference, had in any case moved on. Jason Pontin, evidently chastened by angry readers' responses to his treatment of de Grey, had agreed to support a cash prize for any biologists who could convince a neutral panel of scientists of the falsity of the SENS ideas. By the time we gathered in Atlanta, nobody had yet come forward, clear evidence for the immortalists that de Grey was right and the EMBO signatories and *TR* were wrong.

No layman like myself can hope or even dare to adjudicate in this very bitter contest. In fact, I don't think *anybody* could honestly adjudicate. I say this because, at Atlanta, it became clear, as it had become clear many times before, that the science that forms the basis of this conflict is in flux. Repeatedly, as I have struggled to understand the science that may lead to massive increases in human longevity, I have slumped into depression, concluding that I am just not smart enough. But then, an e-mail or a phone call later, I realise that it's not me, it's the science. It is riddled with contradictions and disagreements. There is neither an overarching theory of ageing, nor is there any consensus about the detailed working of the process and there is certainly nothing like a common view of what approaches might be used. De Grey, as the EMBO signatories must know perfectly well, may be right. Indeed, given our ignorance of the fundamental science involved, his engineering approach may be the only practical way forward and, if we regard the 100,000 who die daily of ageing as a preventable catastrophe, then it also may be seen as the only morally respectable approach.

And so, at the Georgia Tech Conference Center, we had a lawyer, Martine Rothblatt, explaining why even transhumanism – going beyond our biological condition – may not be enough. She wants to see *transbemanism*. The ordinary, biological entity has genes. Richard Dawkins then suggested there may be 'memes', units of cultural transmission, ideas that spread, like genes, through populations. Rothblatt believes we should now think in terms of 'bemes', units of being, so as to include the intelligent computers that will guide us to immortality.

James Hughes, a sociologist from the World Transhumanist Association, attacks the bioconservatives and the Christian Right in the name of 'what we have the potential to become through reason'. Brad Mellon, a Christian theologian, says we must get beyond right-wingers and left-wingers and become 'upwingers'. Eliezer Yudkowsky of the Singularity Institute for Artificial Intelligence shows a slide of a graveyard and asks, 'Are you as tired of this as I am?' Ben Goertzel of Novamente points out that we eat lower animals, we don't want Martine Rothblatt's transbemans eating us. Max More, founder of the Extropy Institute, gives a lecture on how to persuade doubters of the virtues of pursuing immortality. The bouncy 'certified financial planner' Rudi Hoffman, who wears a T-shirt that asks: 'May I bid on your cryonics life insurance?', tells the conference that 'it would be insane not to hit the "save" key on you and your life'.

The passion is obvious, but what lies beyond this passion is The Plan. The Plan is not just immortality, it is a new world of which immortality, though essential, is just one aspect. It is a world in which we shall have gone beyond all the limitations – biological, legal, political, intellectual, financial – of this one. It is the pursuit of the new frontier, not space but time. To the immortalists, a future in which they do not exist has become a personal affront.

The future ennervates but also inspires. Like the deserts and prairies of the West, it demands occupation. And it will be occupied. These people don't just think it's going to happen, they *know* it's going to happen and they want to be ready with the right laws and the right attitudes. Their campaign is, therefore, not to make it happen, but to make it happen as quickly as possible. Lives, lots of them, are at stake. And the Atlanta Braves are galloping to the rescue.

2

The Eternal Thing in Man

The Programme

So why is there suddenly such a thing as the Immortality Institute? Because of a conceptual change in our understanding of the human body. This change is simple. For years – perhaps for all of human history – we assumed that people were programmed to die. Then, over a period of decades, this assumption began to crumble. Finally, in 1977, we found a coherent reason to stop believing in the death programme. This may be wrong – all science is provisional – but, for the moment, the consensus is that there is no death programme and it is this consensus that fires the immortalists.

Belief in such a programme is reasonable enough; indeed, in the face of the facts, it seems undeniable. Everybody dies. We didn't ask to be born, but, once we are, we must die. Why this happens may be open to debate; but that it happens is obvious. It seems natural to assume that it is meant to happen either because God decrees it or because, like everything else in the world, we are worn down by time. It seems natural to assume that the price of life is death, that, in contemporary terms, there is something like a 'death gene' that terminates us when our time comes. Some live longer than others, some age slower and some never seem to suffer illness, but none evades death. Our obsolescence is plainly planned.

The success of modern health technologies provides further evidence of this planning. Medicine, sanitation and all the comforts of civilisation have lengthened our lives to the point where almost everybody experiences old age. People certainly age at different rates, but the same things happen to everybody. Skin wrinkles, strength ebbs, joints stiffen, vision and hearing fade and memory falters. These are clear steps on the road to oblivion. Again, it seems, this must all be one, more or less linear, process, a programmed descent to the grave.

What follows is the story of how this insight was overturned. However, there can be no exact conclusion to this story. The possibility that there is, indeed, a programme remains. Recent research found that knocking out a gene called daf-2 made worms, flies and mice live longer. Some have suggested that this must be the switch that turns on the ageing programme. There is no firm evidence that this is the case – the gene may just incidentally affect ageing. But, even if it is the programme, the immortalists need not despair. If it can simply be knocked out, then lifespan can be very simply extended in everybody.

The Love of a Step-Mother

Further evidence for the intuitively obvious view that there is a programme came in 1859 when Charles Darwin published *On the Origin of Species by Means of Natural Selection, or the Preservation of Favoured Races in the Struggle for Life*. Darwin's insight was simple. When animals or plants reproduce, mistakes – mutations – sometimes occur. Normally these mistakes are of no benefit, but occasionally they are. An organism possessed of a beneficial mutation will do better than other members of its species in a given environment. Some, most or perhaps all of its offspring would inherit the advantage and they, in turn, would be better adapted to their circumstances as a result. In time the species as a whole would change so that the entire population possessed the beneficial mutation. Extrapolated throughout all living history from the first replicating molecule to man, natural selection seems to have the power to explain how the whole variety of life on earth emerged. It is a clear, material process which, given enormous amounts of time, could explain the development of all the complexities of life.

Darwin ended his book by insisting that there was 'grandeur' in this view of life. He did so, defensively, aware of the threat his theory posed to religion. Natural selection seemed to *require* us to die. In fact, the whole structure of Darwinist thought is built on death. Less successful organisms had to die if more successful ones were to prosper. Death was the price of failure. Death cut down those individuals that could not compete. Eventually, of course, it cut down all individuals, but the better adapted lived longer and reproduced more. Darwinism, it has been said, is simply a statement that death is non-random.

This confirmed the intuition that death must be programmed. It was death that had accompanied us on our long journey from the primordial swamp. Death that sorted the wheat from the chaff, slowly building complexity, slowly building the human brain, the organ that would be able to reflect on the fact that it too must die. Stop death and you stop life. It was not God to whom we owed a death, it was Darwin.

It has been said that Darwinism justified atheism. Prior to Darwin, the best possible proof for the existence of God was

the variety and complexity of life. But, since neither Darwin
nor any of his successors have provided a convincing view of
how the whole replication got under way in the first place,
there remains a place for God as the creator, if not of species,
then at least of replication. In fact, it is much more persuasive
to say that Darwin justified death. The answer to the question
'Why must I die?' is, in Darwinian terms, clear. You must die
because it is the price you pay for life, just as all other creatures have died to make way for succeeding generations and
to continue along the path of increasing complexity. Even if
evolution stops with humanity, the price of being human
remains death.

This idea may seem grim but it has its consolations
because, like any religion, it places individuals within a larger
system. The theologian John Bowker is the most cogent
advocate of this view. He has suggested that, after Darwin,
both science and religion now draw the same conclusions.

> . . . first, in rejecting the view that we are trivial and of little
> worth because the universe is so immense and because its
> processes include randomness and chance. . .; and, second,
> in affirming the high value of death as the necessary con-
> dition of life. Both, in their different languages, are saying
> the same thing: it is not possible to have life on any other
> terms than those of death; but where you *do* have death,
> there immediately you have the possibility of life.

As a result, we can make 'of our lives a living sacrifice, a positive acceptance and affirmation on behalf of others that there
are no other terms on which we can have life and live; that we
must grasp death with gratitude, because without it we
cannot grasp anything'. If we celebrate life, we must also celebrate death, the giver of life.

This is of little consolation if the only comfort you can

imagine lies in the perpetuation of yourself. There is no personal immortality on offer here, only the knowledge that, in dying, you are fulfilling the destiny implicit not just in your own birth but in the first successfully replicating molecule. Your 'me' is a fragment of flotsam on the ocean of life. It would mean nothing to that ocean if had you never existed and it certainly means nothing that you do exist. As Miguel de Unamuno cuttingly remarks, quoting Leopardi, nature 'gives us life like a mother, but loves us like a step-mother'. On the other hand, you are part of a newly perceived and understood whole. The ocean made you and to the ocean you shall return.

But, it turns out, not necessarily.

Immortality: The First Glimpse

Missing from Darwin had been any theory of the original replicator, but also Darwin had no idea how the process of inheritance worked. He saw that characteristics must be preserved down the generations but he had no inkling of the mechanism. Mutations could only be effective if they were experiments conducted against a very stable background of inheritance. But what was that background? In fact, almost at exactly the same time that Darwin published *On the Origin of Species*, an Austrian monk, Gregor Mendel, had begun to solve this problem by experimenting with pea plants. He discovered that there were discrete units – what we would now call genes – passed down from generation to generation. In other words, reproduction did not involve, as Darwin had once thought, a simple mixing of parental characteristics. Rather, there was a distinct, mathematically exact transmission of heritable units.

Mendel lived and died in obscurity and his work was not to be discovered by the scientific establishment until 1900,

sixteen years after his death. The central figure in the process
that led to the resurrection of Mendel was the German biologist August Weissman. He had a very simple insight that
was, ultimately, to create the contemporary hope of medical
immortality.

The starting point for this insight was the final refutation
of the work of Jean Baptiste de Lamarck, the French natural-
ist. Lamarck was a crucial figure because, as Darwin
acknowledged, he suggested that species developed according
to law, not divine intervention. But Lamarck's law was that
species developed by inheriting characteristics acquired in
life. So – for some reason, this example is the one always
used – a giraffe stretches its neck to reach leaves on trees and
this lengthened neck is passed on to its offspring. This con-
flicted with Darwinism's requirement of chance mutations as
the driver of change. Nevertheless, it was not immediately
clear that Lamarck was wrong and Darwin was right.
Weissman settled the matter by cutting the tails off successive
generations of mice. By the twenty-second generation mice
with tails were still being born of tail-less parents. Nothing
was changed by the repeated amputations.

Or, rather, something remained obdurately unchanged.
Whatever insults the parent mice endured in life, their offspring were always created anew. The message, the plan, the
blueprint, the scheme of a new and perfect mouse was preserved intact. And so, in Weissman's terms, the organism
consisted of germ cells – the carriers of the blueprint – and
somatic cells – the remaining cells of the body. This was his
germ plasm theory. The germ cells were protected from any
abuse to the somatic cells. They were the precious cargo
within the battered vessel of the body. Lamarck was thus
wrong, reproduction was unaffected by the life of the somatic
cells, and Darwin, once we allow for the fact that chance
mutations can arise in the germ cells, was right. (This is not

absolutely the case. Radiation, for example, is an external influence that can affect the germ cells. But such exceptions are minor breaches of what is a very clear law.)

This distinction between the immortal cells of reproduction and the mortal ones of the individual life has proved almost as influential an insight as Darwinism itself. It has an obvious symmetry with the religious idea of the immortal soul encased in the mortal body, though the 'soul' in this case is emphatically not the self, which dies with the body.

The poet and novelist Thomas Hardy tried to derive consolation from the apparent immortality of our inherited characteristics in 'Heredity':

> The years-heired feature that can
> In curve and voice and eye
> Despise the human span
> Of durance – that is I;
> The eternal thing in man,
> That heeds no call to die.

And Sigmund Freud was drawn to the apparent symmetry of cellular immortality and personal mortality. His own belief in the centrality of human sexuality to the construction of the various layers of the self was derived from the Darwinian model that had placed reproduction at the centre of a human identity defined by its biology. That was *eros*. But Freud came to be convinced of the incompleteness of that model and added *thanatos*, a drive towards death that explained otherwise wholly irrational catastrophes like the slaughter during the First World War. Thus Freud embedded the Weissmanian insight deep inside our identities. The germ cells drove us towards sex and reproduction; the somatic cells drove us towards death. Our desire and our demise were two sides of the same biological coin.

But, strictly in terms of the science of biology, Weissman had formalised the central idea of Darwinism, that all living things are related and all descend from the same initial replicator. Our germ cells are our link to every other living thing. Our somatic cells are just the chance products of the germ cells brought about by the meeting of our parents. They are mortal and subject to decay.

'Death occurs', said Weissman, 'because a worn out tissue cannot forever renew itself.'

But this famous quotation contains the shadow of a contradiction. For, if the somatic cells were mortal, that must mean that the germs cells were *immortal*, that there was, therefore, something that did not wear out. This is not strictly a contradiction because what survives of the germ cells is not tissue, but the information contained in the DNA. Nevertheless, Weissman was the first person to use the word 'immortal' about cells. Something living, something inside us was immortal, it had existed as long as there had been life. Individuals are mortal; life is not. There was something eternal in man.

Not Quite Death in Baltimore

A tantalising possibility had been born, the possibility of immortal, living entities. In fact, we had always known about such entities and, as life expectancies increased in the twentieth century, we came to know them even better because they killed us in ever greater numbers. Cancer is immortal.

Henrietta Lacks was born in 1920 in Clover, Virginia, a tobacco and cotton town. Like almost everybody else in Clover, Henrietta was black and poor and, also like everybody else, she came from a large family. Indeed, her family was so big that part of Clover was known as Lacks Town. Henrietta joined this family by marrying David Lacks and, in

1942, they travelled north to Baltimore, looking for work. Baltimore was booming because ships had to be built for the war effort and David got a job with Bethlehem Steel at Sparrow's Point on the waterfront. Fortuitously, for this story, Baltimore was also the home of Johns Hopkins Hospital, one of the greatest medical institutions in the world.

David and Henrietta had five children and lived in Turner Station, a suburb across the Patapsco River estuary from Sparrow's Point. Every summer she went back to Clover and, throughout the year, she put up visitors from the south. She seems to have been a happy, balanced person. The one big shadow in her life was the epilepsy of her eldest daughter, Elsie.

But then, in January 1951, Henrietta noticed she was bleeding from her vagina. On the 1st of February she went to the women's clinic of Johns Hopkins Hospital. The gynaecologist, Dr Howard Jones, found an inch-wide lobe of tissue on her cervix. But it did not look like cervical cancer. This tumour was more vigorous and better supplied with blood vessels than anything Dr Jones had seen before. Puzzled, he had Henrietta tested for syphilis. The test was negative. So Dr Jones cut off a section of the lump to be examined by a pathologist and Henrietta was told that same day that she had cervical cancer.

There were only two treatments available at the time – surgery and radiation. Jones went for the latter and a surgeon stitched a tube containing radium capsules to her cervix. Twenty-four hours later he removed the tube, recording that 'the patient feels quite well tonight'. She could have been fine. Radium had a good record against cervical cancer – most patients were still alive five years after therapy. Henrietta went home to wait. But what she did not know, what nobody in her family was to know for another twenty-five years, was that the surgeon had cut one normal piece of tissue and one cancerous from Henrietta and sent them to Dr George Gey, a researcher at the Johns Hopkins medical school.

Gey, like many others, had been trying to cultivate human cell lines in the laboratory. He had, so far, been unsuccessful but there was something odd about Henrietta's tumour. Once placed in Gey's culturing medium, it grew and grew. This was good news for science, but the vigour of the cancer was bad news for Henrietta. She died on 4 October 1951. Gey concealed Henrietta's identity by calling the cell line HeLa. He started sending samples all over the world. He gave them away free and his parcels became known as 'helagrams'. The HeLa line became a laboratory gold standard around the world.

Unlike most cancerous cells, they were virtually normal and thus superb study specimens. HeLa was involved in the study of at least 174 different human genes and instrumental in the development of the polio virus. HeLa also went into space on board the Discovery XVII satellite. The cells remain in use and it is now thought that the total of HeLa in the world weighs more than Henrietta did when she was alive.

But the sheer potency of the cells also had the effect of hindering scientific research. In a lab, HeLa cells are perfectly capable of infecting other cultures. As result, scientists may think they are working on one type of cell when they are actually working on HeLa. Lines of cells from the Soviet Union, said to be from Caucasians, turned out to be HeLa, a discovery that at once discredited the Soviet belief that these lines revealed a viral cause for cancer. In 1968 it became clear that twenty-four out of thirty-four cell lines at the US central cell bank, the American Type Culture Collection, all of which were supposed to be different, were, in fact, HeLa.

Finally, the name of the donor of the cells was revealed and Henrietta became famous. Writing an article for the *Sunday*

Times magazine about this story some years ago, I visited Turner Station and met her relatives and friends. The revelation of Henrietta's posthumous role had inspired conflicting emotions. Some were angry, feeling the family was owed compensation by Johns Hopkins and that the original use of the cells had been underhand. In fact, Johns Hopkins made no money from the cells. Others expressed pride at the contribution Henrietta's cells had made to medical research. She was, they said, a heroine of the poor blacks who moved from Virginia to Baltimore, of, indeed, all black Americans. In truth, of course, she did nothing but contract cancer. But identity in America is an issue that tends to have access to all areas.

But all of that is trivial next to one reaction, one best expressed by her friend Sadie Sturdivant. They used to go to the Adams Lounge together and drink cocktails. How, I asked Sadie, did she feel when she heard about the trillions of Henrietta's cells still alive around the world.

'I was shocked. They'd taken something out of her and it was still living. Sometimes when I think about that it makes me feel a little shakey. I never knowed they could live like that. When you sit back and think about that a kind of cold chill go over you. What it really mean?'

It means different things on either side of the cultural gulf that divides poor, uneducated people from the intellectual grandeur of Johns Hopkins. When it comes to Henrietta's cells, for example, the word 'living' means to the Johns Hopkins scientists merely that they have retained their biochemical integrity and capacity to replicate themselves. To the family and Sadie, it means that some part of their mother is still alive, that, in some way, she survived the appalling cancer that struck back in 1951. She has attained some shadowy kind of immortality.

Of course, Johns Hopkins is right. We cannot talk to these

cells as if they were Henrietta. Even if we could produce a clone of Henrietta from the massive supplies of her DNA now available, it would not be the Henrietta that moved from Virginia to Baltimore, married David and had five children, acquiring memories along the way. Henrietta Lacks still died on 4 October 1951.

And yet the feeling that, somehow, she did not completely die is both ancient, intuitively potent and, in one narrow scientific sense, correct. From Weissman's insight, we know that we are chance emanations of the germ plasm. That emanation consists, initially, of our unique genetic structure, the particular combination of our parent's DNA. As we develop, we become even more individualised by environment and experience. In Henrietta's case, this process of individualisation included a mutation in chromosome 11 of one of her cells, the deletion of a tumour-suppressor gene that allowed that particular cell to become cancerous. Scientists must now agree that, following Darwin and Weissman, our bodies are part mortal and part immortal. But the immortal part normally survives in our offspring. In Henrietta's case it survives in the cells. Sadie Sturdivant's intuition that this extraordinary fact must mean something, that it must ask a question, is absolutely correct.

'What it really mean?'

A Giant Rooster and the Death Clock

Alexis Carrel was a French biologist who worked in New York. In 1912 he put a fragment of the heart of a chicken embyro in a growth medium. The cells divided and the fragment grew in size. The cells were still dividing thirty-five years later. These were not cancer cells and not germ cells, they were somatic cells. And yet they appeared to be immortal. For almost fifty years, scientists were convinced that

Carrel's chick heart had refuted Weissman's conviction that somatic cells were mortal.

The experiment made headlines. In 1921 the *World* newspaper in New York claimed the total mass of cells produced would have made 'a rooster . . . big enough to cross the Atlantic in a stride'. As in the case of Henrietta Lacks, there was confusion about the difference between a mass of cells and a complete organism. Furthermore, the idea of this constantly expanding, living blob probably inspired a good deal of science fiction imagery.

The experiment had profound scientific implications. It suggested that somatic cells were immortal but could only become so when placed in ideal but artificial conditions. For fifty years cell biologists accepted this as proven beyond doubt. This raised the question: what made cells die in the body? The answer to that question should have provided the answer to why we age and die. Hormones, material binding cells together, cosmic rays were all put in the dock accused of cell-murder. The living cell had become what the newborn child is to the romantic imagination, an object of perfection doomed to be corrupted by its society/environment, in this case the body itself. Carrel's chick heart seemed to show that immortality was our natural primordial condition. Far from being programmed to die, we were meant to live.

Except that Carrel's experimental procedure was all wrong. In the late fifties, in Philadelphia, Leonard Hayflick discovered his error. While working on populations of human cells, Hayflick noticed that many were dying. And the ones that were dying were those that had divided most often. All the cell lines had been kept with immense care in ideal conditions, so the prevailing dogma was that they should not die. But they did and, not only that, they did not die randomly. They died when they got old. Eventually it became clear that cells died after dividing about fifty times – for perspective, it takes about forty doublings for the fertilised human egg to produce an adult human. Hayflick had discovered cellular ageing.

Carrel's mistake lay in his technique. He used chick embyro extract to fix his heart to the culture vessel. Cells had supposedly been removed from this extract, but, in fact, they hadn't. So every time tissue was glued down, cells were added. Carrel was constantly reseeding his population. It was not immortal at all.

The limit on the number of times somatic cells can double became known as the Hayflick Limit. On the face of it, this seems to be a pretty clear death clock, a point beyond which we cannot take our bodies. For most of us, however, the Hayflick Limit is irrelevant. Fifty doublings is quite enough to give us a very long life and its limitation is only likely to affect us when we are well over a hudred. If it is a death clock, few of us will live to see it stop. It may, however, be the marker of maximum human lifespan. In his book *How and Why We Age*, Hayflick suggested this was about 115. For other scientists, however, there is no such thing. The most recent evidence is that the limit is highly malleable and, therefore, not a death sentence but simply an aspect of the ageing processes of the body.

Nevertheless, Hayflick had destroyed the idea of any natural or primordial immortality in normal somatic cells. But the immortality of germ and cancer cells, and, therefore, the possibility of immortal life, remained intact.

Killer Genes

One thing that struck Hayflick was the utter futility of the ageing process. He wrote:

After performing the miracles that take us from conception to birth, and then to sexual maturation and adulthood, nature chose not to devise what would seem to be a more elementary mechanism to simply maintain those miracles forever. This insight has puzzled biogerontologists for decades.

Virtually all biological events from conception to maturity seem to have a purpose, but aging does not. It is not obvious why aging should occur.

Ageing seems so normal and pervasive a phenomena that this observation may seem odd. Ageing, obviously, is the body running downhill. There is no reason why it should have a purpose any more than a bald car tyre or a worn-out carpet should have a purpose. It is just wear and tear. But, as Hayflick also points out, '. . . time itself produces no biological effects. Events occur in time but not because of its passage.' The tyre is bald because it has been used in a particular way, not because it is old. Left unused, its tread would be intact after centuries. Time itself is not the enemy, events are the enemy. In the words of Indiana Jones, 'It's not the years, honey, it's the mileage.' This is a surprisingly exact biological observation. There is nothing about duration itself that ages us. Germ lines and cancer cells prove that biological mechanisms can maintain themselves forever. Indeed, some complete organisms make the same point or at least we think they do. Freshwater hydra appear to be immortal and, it is thought, some fish simply grow and grow without ever showing signs of age. There is a creosote bush in the American desert that is thought to be 10,000 years old and the species itself may well be immortal. It is obviously hard to be sure about any of this as that would require an infinite amount of time spent watching fish or bushes.

The problem with ageing, however, is that, in spite of its familiarity, it is an extremely difficult to define. Exact or even reasonably precise biological markers for ageing – effectively an internal odometer that gave comparable readings in different people – have proved hard to find. Not only do different people age at different rates, but also different parts of the same person age at different rates. I recently spoke to a ninety-five-year-old woman. She certainly looked her age, but her mind was as sharp and as clear as a forty-year-old's. Equally, I have met seventy-five-year-olds who couldn't remember from moment to moment what they were talking about and sixty-year-olds who look no older than forty-five. Most attempts to find one, clear ageing marker have failed. This is a problem for the view that death is programmed. If it were, surely we could see some consistency in the working out of that programme rather than this random stumble into the grave.

Curiously, however, one very precise definition of ageing has emerged that does not involve the body at all. In the early nineteenth century, statistical data about the human population was just becoming widely available. An English actuary, Benjamin Gompertz, studied death rates and made the weird discovery that, after the age of thirty, the likelihood of any individual dying doubled every eight years. The finding was precise enough to lay the foundations of the life-insurance industry. The only reason you can buy life insurance at all is that the companies know with a remarkable degree of precision what the death rates will be in any given population.

After Gompertz, it became clear that ageing is best defined, not as a physical condition, but as a probability. This is the formulation of the biologist John Maynard Smith – 'Ageing is a progressive, generalised impairment of function resulting in an increasing probability of death.' A hydra – if it is immortal – or a fish – if it is immortal – has a body that stays the same through time. Its probability of dying, therefore, is constant throughout its life. (Even if it is immortal in this sense, it will eventually die because this probability is finite. One day a rock will crush the hydra or a shark will eat the fish.) On the other hand, animals that age have a daily increasing probability of dying. I am more likely to die today than I was yesterday and twice as likely as I was eight years ago.

The importance of this definition is that it is statistical. Ageing is defined by an abstraction, a probability, rather than by a physical marker. This, in turn, points to what ageing ultimately is now seen to be – not the result of programmed internal decline but of random insult. But I shall return to this very soon.

In the fifties two scientists – Sir Peter Medawar in Britain and George Williams in the US – considered the idea of errors as the source of ageing. This is a familiar concept. Cars age, for example, because errors occur in the form of corrosion, damaged or worn-out parts and so on. The body is somewhat different in that it has sophisticated error correction processes. But errors do occur in the replication of DNA. These can produce errors in protein production. Such errors will be rare and random but will, over time, steadily accumulate. Ageing might be seen as the progressive accumulation of such errors.

Medawar and Williams developed this possibility into the concept of 'antagonistic pleiotropy'. Pleiotropy is the ability of genes to have two completely different functions. Thus, famously, the gene for sickle-cell anaemia provides some protection against malaria. It is beneficial to have one copy of this gene as it will make you less likely to contract malaria, but catastrophic to have two because you will contract sickle-cell anaemia. Medawar and Williams, in slightly different ways, postulated that there may be genes that are good early in life and bad in later life. Ideally, these genes should remain beneficial until after reproductive maturity, after which nature – our stepmother – loses all interest in us. It may be the case that the gene for Huntington's chorea is a very clear example. If you have this gene, you will certainly contract the disease, but not until middle age. In other words, it kicks in after sexual maturity. Equally, calcium is good for children, bad for adults. Evolution has left us with a life of two halves.

There are two ways of looking at this. Either good, beneficial genes in youth turn bad in old and middle age. Or the body successfully controls the malign effects of bad genes for a time, but then loses its grip and the bad genes take over. In both cases there is an age barrier, a moment when the body seems to topple over into decline. The possibility of a programmed death remains – good genes turning bad could be just such a programme – but it has been weakened. Rather what we seem to have now is a decline made statistically certain by the accumulation of random damage. The problem with this is that it still doesn't answer Hayflick's question: what is the purpose of ageing? In natural selection, almost everything must have a clear, evolutionary purpose and certainly something as radical and prevalent as ageing should be explicable in evolutionary terms. In fact, as with so many big questions, the answer is only found when we stop asking.

In Tom Kirkwood's Bath

In 1977, in his bath, in Mill Hill, London, Tom Kirkwood had an idea. He was twenty-five at the time and an intellectual hybrid. His Cambridge degree was in mathematics and he had an Oxford higher degree in statistics, but he had always been drawn to biology. In 1973 he began work at the National Institute for Biological Standards and Control in London. There he developed the International Normalised Ratio which measures the coagulability of blood. INR appears on hospital patients' charts all over the world. The sight of the letters still makes him proud.

At some point, he remembers a conversation in a lift with

a scientist about how cells age. This interested him and, by 1975, he had published two papers on the subject of ageing. He thought about this for another two years and then, in his bath, realised why humans age. In a nutshell: they age because, in nature, almost nothing ever does.

We don't see this because we are blinded by the comforts of civilisation and modernity. We see humans and certain animals – our pets, farm animals – age and we even see plants wither and die in our gardens. But all of these organisms are living highly protected lives. In the wild, they are exposed to constant assault and engaged in a perpetual struggle for survival. As a result, they die much younger than ourselves or our domesticated animals. The proportion that actually age is very small. In nature, it is normal to be cut down in the prime of life.

Kirkwood is the central figure in this story for several reasons. First, he condensed the several strands of thought about ageing, specifically the Medawar–Williams development of the error theory. Indeed, scientists who feel that Kirkwood has been given too much credit – backstabbing is routine in this highly competitive world – argue that his insight amounts to no more than 'a worked example of antagonistic pleiotropy'. This requires translation into English. Basically, the argument is that Kirkwood has added nothing new to the insights of Medawar and Williams. All he has done is apply their insights in an evolutionary context. He has done nothing more than conduct an experiment based on the theory. Personally, I think this a pretty obvious example of professional jealousy. As I shall explain, the evolutionary context changes everything in ways that the basic theory could not.

Kirkwood is also central because he is routinely cited as the inspirer of the new longevity/immortality movement. He demonstrated not only that the body is not programmed to die but also why it is not so programmed. The body is,

therefore, fixable. Furthermore, Kirkwood is a contemporary – for me, almost an exact one – and his experiences and
attitudes with regard to ageing and death are a mirror of our
own. He is diffident about this, but the more I spoke to him,
the more it became clear that the confusions of contemporary
secularity about ageing and dying are implicit in his life and
work.

He is now fifty-four and co-director of the Institute for
Ageing and Health at Newcastle University. He looks easy to
get on with and he is. He also looks well. His hair is still dark
and, though he is a little paunchy, it is within healthy limits.
He wears a university tie because it saves difficult choices in
the morning. We both have a feeling we have met before.
But, later, I decide this is because his face is similar to that of
the writer Robert Harris. I tell him this and he remarks that
he has often noticed the way human faces fall into types,
suggesting a limited range of genetic variation. I had noticed
the same thing but assumed I was imagining it.

His office in the new Henry Wellcome Laboratory for
Biogerontology Research at Newcastle General Hospital is
full of papers, files, books, a bike and a small, disconnected
electronic keyboard, but it is not a mess. I feel he knows
where everything is. There is also a precision about the way
he responds to my arrival. It is lunchtime and he walks me
briskly round the hospital grounds to a café. I am alarmed. It
looks noisy and uncomfortable. But we are merely there to
buy our sandwiches – egg and beef, both high cholesterol
choices, a fact of some significance, I shall later discover –
and then return to his office. There he provides coffee and,
for some reason, a cone-shaped Ukrainian chocolate. We
crouch round a small table, moving papers to accommodate
our lunches.

He was born in South Africa, one of six children.
Mathematically, he says, he is as near to being the middle of

six as it is possible to be because two of the later children were twins. It is a neat thought that is very characteristic of the man. Later he was to have twins of his own, a boy and a girl.

'Ah,' he says after a pause, 'you passed the test, you did not ask if they were identical.'

Identical twins must, of course, be of the same sex, yet apparently many people still ask if his boy and girl are identical. He noticed that I did not. Again, very characteristic.

This is a man who watches the world closely for signs, indications of order, clues. Faces are a sign of limited genetic variation; twins somehow modify the evenness of the number six; people do not grasp the concept of the naturally cloned genome that produces identical twins. On top of that, his office is complex but organised, like life. Kirkwood had to be like this to see what he saw in the bath.

The family moved to Britain when he was four, his father having been appalled by government-sanctioned racism. They lived in Oxford and Kirkwood was sent to a very traditional primary school where he was taught Latin and Greek but almost no science. Luckily for him, this changed in his secondary school. He had a rare talent for maths.

'In a deep sense, I've got a sort of intuitive connection with maths, but I've also always been passionately interested in biology, forever paddling around in streams.'

They went back to live in his mother's home country – Rhodesia, now Zimbabwe – for a year when Kirkwood was thirteen. At school there, he was so far ahead of the other pupils that he had to be moved to successively higher years. He spent his spare time reading books and watching termites build their nests. Returning to England, he went on to Cambridge to take maths as a degree.

While studying statistics, he learned of the uses of mathematics in biology. The structure of the DNA molecule had been deciphered by Watson and Crick in 1953. This structure had two crucial attributes: its double-helix shape suggest how organisms might replicate and the four nucleotide bases that bridge the twin spirals indicate how genetic information might be encoded. As the implications of the discovery were worked out, it became clear that there was a computer-like system at the heart of life. This system was based on the four nucleotide 'digits' that made up the genes that specified the proteins necessary to construct living things. In fact, this system has proved to be far more complex than first thought and not very much like a computer. Nevertheless, the deciphering of DNA and the subsequent rise of the discipline of molecular biology meant that mathematics had been brought decisively into biology. Indeed, the subject was transformed. Where once biology had been 'horizontal' – an acquisition of disparate data – it now became, like mathematics, 'vertical' – a systematic construction of a theoretical model of life processes.

Kirkwood fully understood this when he read John Kendrew's *The Thread of Life: An Introduction to Molecular Biology*. The two obsessions of his own life – mathematics and biology – now turned out to be the two disciplines at the centre of the most creative science of the age. In addition, his order-seeking personality had found an endorsement in nature.

'I found it so exciting that living systems had this underpinning order. It was just wonderful.'

Ageing and dying were the particular subjects he studied. He gently resists any suggestion that anything in his personality drew him to these areas.

'I can't precisely say what intrigued me. I suppose it was the mysterious nature of the process. It was a universal process going on in all of us but we knew remarkably little about it. From a biological perspective it was highly complicated . . . It appealed to the mathematician in me. Probably there is a deeper emotional resonance, though it wasn't obvious to me at the time. It's become a bit more obvious as I've broadened my activity.'

Death, he says, 'didn't loom large on my radar' in childhood. But there was one evidently traumatic incident. When he was sixteen, his best friend was a boy called Richard. One day Richard was watching a documentary on television on ageing called, as Kirkwood recalls, 'When I'm 64'. As the programme ended, Richard said, 'I hope I never end up like that.' He went out for a run round the block and never returned. He had died of a heart attack. His family had a history of hypercholesterolemia.

Kirkwood says he doesn't feel there was any connection between that loss and his subsequent interest in ageing. But the aftermath of Richard's death clearly left a mark on his imagination. The family weakness had struck several times. Richard's father had died young and his brother had died very early.

'Richard's mother was a wonderful woman, but I think possibly she had become quite hardened to loss. He was cremated and I think I felt a sense of the lack of an obvious place to go to experience grief. There's something to be said for a grave and a headstone . . . I was conscious then that I would have liked the opportunity for a leave-taking. I think it's important. We've lost that capacity to share in and support the end of life.'

It looks as though, even if the incident did not inspire Kirkwood's later preoccupations, it deepened them. The very fact that he had not been exposed to much death in childhood makes Richard's story all the more stark and memorable. It is also significant what conclusions the incident drew from him. Many, inspired by the prospect of defeating death scientifically, take the death of someone close to them as a spur to their efforts. But Kirkwood's response is to nurture a respect for death. Similarly, he resists the idea that his current work is anything to do with pursuing immortality.

'I disagree with life extensionists. I think it's entirely wrong. I get quite angry with the emphasis that is being placed on life extension as the benefit we seek to derive from this research. We've extended life quite a lot over the last hundred years so the issue for the vast majority of older people is the quality of life they have in those extra years. I think it's immoral to steer the discussion to the extension of life when we've got real old people in real difficulty.'

Medicine, he believes, has always had difficulties with this.

'The thing that's impelled the increase in life expectancy has been the desire to prevent death. We've been spectacularly successful in pursuing that to the extent that we have doubled life expectancy in the last 200 years ... We want to prevent death, don't we? But ageing, illness and death are part of the reason why, for many doctors, issues related to the end of life and ageing are difficult to accommodate as they run counter to the whole motivation structure, the intellectual structure and, for so many doctors, ageing and death are proof of failure.'

This is a crucial point. La Rochefoucauld said looking directly at death was like staring at the sun. We spend most of our lives trying not to look, fearing we shall be blinded. Kirkwood's point is that the medical profession is no different, they run away from death. And so, in spite of the fact that defeating death is what, above all else, they do, they prefer not to consider the inevitable failure of this project. The study of ageing and dying has, therefore, been seen as not quite respectable, possibly disgusting or even risible. Hayflick made the same point in 1994: 'For many scientists, ageism is coupled with the belief that growing old is intractable, an absolute certainty that is best ignored. As recently as fifteen years ago, the few researchers working in the field of ageing were sometimes derided or ridiculed by fellow scientists.'

Apart from Kirkwood and Hayflick, many others tell this same story. In one sense this medical fear of, horror at or avoidance of the study of ageing and death is the scientific correlative of the denial of death defined by Geoffrey Gorer and subsequently taken up by Philippe Aries. Both represent a crisis of secularity, an inability to provide rites, words or a context for a process that represents an absolutely unavoidable affront to our dreams of progress and self-actualisation. The relative's despair at finding the right words at the bedside is the same as the jaunty doctor's refusal to countenance a failure he knows is inevitable. One of the unarguably beneficial side-effects of the new pursuit of immortality is that it has opened up an entirely new area of medical research. Whatever this achieves in terms of human longevity, it should certainly help alleviate the sufferings of the old, sufferings brought on by the previous triumphs of medicine and social policy in extending human life.

The incident of Richard's death and his cremation dramatised, for Kirkwood, the peculiarly modern, secular confusion into which we have sunk on the subject of death. Kirkwood's mathematical imagination discovered in molecular biology a complex discipline that offered tantalising possibilities of resolution. In Darwinism, there was, of course, an over-arching theory but there was no one way of tying any individual phenomenon into the theory. In the case of ageing, here was a phenomenon that was both obvious and universal but which, on closer inspection, seemed to evade any rational explanation in Darwinian or, indeed, any other terms. Dying itself might be seen as a Darwinian necessity in that it made way for future generations to improve the species. But ageing made no obvious sense. If everything was a Darwinian process, what possible naturally selective pressure required our skin to wrinkle, our eyesight to fade, our hearing to lose its acuity, our memory to falter, our bones to thin, our muscles to shrink and our arteries to harden? Medawar and Williams had shown how this might happen, but not why.

And then Kirkwood took his bath. The issue that led to the resolution of all this was error suppression. One of the most startling things about life on earth is its persistence in the face of very adverse conditions. It is one thing to say that somehow certain molecules in the warm soup of primeval earth accidentally stumbled upon a system of replication which, as soon as it was up and running, was subject to the creative force of natural selection. It is quite another thing to say that this system will manage to protect itself for millennia against dissolution and fragmentation. Most obviously, there is the problem not just of replicating oneself, but also of replicating oneself with almost absolute accuracy. Some degree of error is permissible – indeed, it is necessary if natural selection is to work at all – but, on the whole, errors in replication are catastrophic. What those first molecules needed, therefore, was a near perfect system of error suppression.

Plainly, if we assume that the first successful replications happened by chance, then we know that subsequent ones were protected by natural selection. Only the best replicators would survive to replicate. Subsequent generations, therefore, would be the product of the best. This would put a constant pressure on the replication process to improve itself, to protect itself from decay and dissolution. Part of this protection would involve ensuring that the entire system – both replicating machinery and the body that carried it – was efficient and tough and enough to reach the point of replication. But, crucially, the replicating system itself would require the most protection as it would outlast the individual body to live on in the next generation.

The work of Medawar and Williams emphasised the importance of this. Plainly the key moment in the process of life is replication or reproduction. As far as natural selection is concerned, that is the only point of the organism. Once reproduction is over, the organism is redundant. Nature has no further use for it. Medawar and Williams saw that this could mean that genes – our modern idea of fundamental replicators – would be configured to produce their most beneficial effects on the organism in the period up to and including its reproductive phase. After that, however, it didn't matter what they did.

This would mean there was no one 'death gene' or trigger of ageing; rather there was simply a progressive build up of errors. These would not happen in a pre-programmed way, but merely by chance. In theory, a human being could evade all this chance damage and avoid ageing completely. In practice, this is impossible, the odds are too heavily stacked against us. Internal errors occur or the environment attacks the organism and it decays and, finally, dies. As the errors increase, genes that were once good for us turn bad. Hence antagonistic pleiotropy.

But this still wasn't quite right. Nature could have produced an organism that simply went on reproducing throughout its entire life. Creating one brief span of reproduction once you have gone to all the trouble of producing an entire organism seems absurdly inefficient. Indeed, one of the more startling things about nature's behaviour is her insane profligacy. Trillions of fantastically complex organisms are produced and then simply discarded. Every living cell is a machine of staggering intricacy and yet each is utterly disposable. Surely, if natural selection works towards greater competitive efficiency, then a better use of resources would be one obvious approach.

Kirkwood saw the answer to this problem in his bath. It is simply that most animals do not get the chance to age. In the wild, they die of starvation, disease or predation long before ageing can happen. Obviously, there are some exceptions.

Creatures at the top of the food chain will be less liable to predation so one might see, for example, an old lion. But lions will be equally susceptible to starvation and disease, so old lions will be a lot rarer than old people in the modern world. Equally, we all know of ancient elephants and tortoises. But, again, these seem to be rarities. The overall picture – and it is this broad, generalised way of life on which evolution must act – is that living in the wild is very dangerous.

The earliest humans, it is thought, had a life expectancy at birth of no more than eighteen. Anything we might regard as a minor disruption to our lives today – flu, a throat infection, a broken limb – would be fatal in the wild. This has been the case since the first replicating molecules emerged. The threats to them would be non-living chaos and disorder, constantly attempting to tear them apart and, eventually, succeeding. But, as life expanded to cover the entire planet, the threats became predators and bacteria. Wild life is constantly in a condition of war. And humans, for most of their time on earth, have lived in the wild.

In that context, it becomes clear that there is absolutely no point in nature producing a long-lived replicator. Its efforts would be in vain. In the wild, any replicator will be lucky to replicate once successfully. Hayflick wondered why nature hadn't taken the obvious step of making her organisms immortal. But there was no point. A Rolls-Royce body would, in the wild, last no longer than a Ford. Nature's most efficient strategy, therefore, would be to put all her efforts into getting its creatures to reproduce. After that, they were surplus to requirements. There could be no selective pressure to improve the condition of a body that had passed its reproductive phase.

There are two stages to nature's strategy: putting maximum effort into protecting the germ line and putting just enough effort into the protection of the soma or body to get it through to reproduction. The important words here are 'just enough'. There is no Darwinian advantage in making bodies that last beyond their reproductive phase. Or, put another way, it is logically impossible for natural selection to sustain bodies into old age as it can only work on the repro-ductive process. Ask natural selection about the purpose of ageing and it would not understand the question.

'Animals in the wild,' says Kirkwood, 'never live long enough to exhibit signs of ageing. That tells you that most animals never need an ageing process . . . You can't evolve through natural selection some process that works in a hypo-thetical age range that is never realised. A lot of people when confronted with that argument go on working incredibly hard to refute it. The reason is that there is, at some level, an emotional need to make sense of a process as universal as ageing.'

One can hardly overstate the significance of this insight, christened by Kirkwood the Disposable Soma Theory. It shifts our perspective in two fundamental ways. First, by drawing attention to the fact that ageing doesn't happen in the wild, the theory transforms our sense of the 'naturalness' of the process. In fact, ageing is almost entirely a product of civilisation. As I said, very early man's life expectancy was probably only about eighteen. That is how long hunter-gatherers could expect to live at birth. As soon as agriculture and the resulting settlements appeared, the figure began to rise. At the time of the Roman Empire, life expectancy is thought to have risen to twenty-two, though for the wealthy with access to food and shelter it would have been much higher. In the Middle Ages in Britain, the figure was thirty-three. But the big increases began at the beginning of the eighteenth century. In the industrialised countries, life expectancy rose from forty to about forty-nine in 1900 and then to around seventy-five or more today. We all live most of our lives on borrowed time, time that our stepmother nature never intended us to have.

'The price we pay for the fact that our social and cultural evolution has outstripped the pace of our biological evolution,' Kirkwood has written, 'is that we experienced ageing to an extent that has probably never occurred in the living world before. We are, as Amercian physician Boyd Eaton has put it, "stone agers in the fast lane".'

When told these figures about life expectancies, people tend to extrapolate what they are familiar with into the past. Thus, they might say that eighteen-year-old hunter gatherers or thirty-three-year-old medieval peasants were old in the same way that eighty-year-olds are said to be old today. This is a mistake. It is true that these age groups in these different eras would have in common a closer proximity to death than the rest of the population. But the eighteen-year-old and the thirty-three-year-old would not share the eighty-year-old's experience of ageing. They would not have the wrinkles, the grey hair or any of the more serious conditions associated with being old because the antagonistic effects of their genes would not yet have occurred. The same point is made by the transformation in the causes of death over time. In 1900 the major cause of death was infectious disease – tuberculosis, pneumonia – today the major causes are cardiovascular diseases – heart attacks, strokes – and cancer. Deaths from the most common infectious killers in 1900 are all but unknown in the wealthiest countries. The point is that, in 1900, most people did not live long enough to experience heart attacks and cancer. Now they do. They live long enough to know old age.

The second shift in perspective caused by the Disposable Soma Theory is even more startling in its implications. If there is no inbuilt mechanism of ageing and dying, no 'death

gene', then all that happens is that we reach a peak of reproductive fitness and then start to die. Natural selection has not
bothered to protect our bodies beyond this peak and so we
gradually succumb to various cellular deteriorations and environmental insults. The uniformity we think we detect in the
ageing process is, in part, an illusion. What is actually happening is that we are afflicted by a series of chance
developments, some of which – say, grey hair – are very likely
to happen, and some of which – say, Parkinson's disease – are
somewhat less likely.

This means that we do not die, we are killed. This changes
everything.

Sheep 6LL3

Lab subject 6LL3, aka Dolly the Sheep, was born on 5 July
1996 and died on 14 February 2003. She was the first clone of
an adult mammalian cell. Geneticists were stunned. One I
spoke to in America soon afterwards had been forced to rush
round to his publishers to make changes to a book just before
printing. He had written that such a procedure was impossible.

Dolly has been much discussed, but all that is necessary is
to understand why geneticists were so shocked by the development. Most adult somatic cells are known to contain all the
DNA – all the genes – necessary for the construction of a complete creature. However, these cells are differentiated according
to the work they must do. So, for example, liver cells have
all the genes turned off except those required to make the
liver work. That turning off process was thought to be irreversible and that was the reason cloning from a differentiated
cell was thought to be impossible. Dolly proved this to be
wrong.

Kirkwood has written of the implications of this. 'What
Dolly has shown is that there is something about germ cells

that can apparently override the ageing of somatic cells. The idea that wear and tear is an inevitable feature of living systems is not a good enough explanation of ageing.'

Dolly was, in fact, the ovine face of the massive extension of our technical capabilities within biology. This is centred on stem cells, undifferentiated cells that retain the ability to become any specialised cell within the body. They were first derived from mouse embryos in the 1980s but, in 1998, it was discovered how to acquire stem cells from human embryos. We can now acquire them from adult tissue. Like Dolly, our ability to retrieve and use stem cells represents a fundamental change in our sense of how far we can go in controlling our biology. A stem cell takes us back to the roots of our biological being. In doing so, it implies that anything is possible, not least immortality.

Weissman has been proved wrong. Turning on all the genes on a somatic cell effectively rejuvenated that cell, turning its clock back to the moment of its creation. Of course, the cell would still be damaged by the ageing it had already endured as a differentiated cell. But the principle had been established that the cells of our body are not necessarily destined to die. And neither, therefore, are we.

Towards the Invisible Death

If, in our imaginations, the human body is programmed to die, the process of ageing and dying is the predestined natural order of things, then disease would be seen as an event that stands outside this process. Infectious diseases, like smallpox or tuberculosis, are obviously invasions from outside our bodily system. Since such infectious diseases were the major causes of death in the human population until the twentieth century, it must have seemed reasonable to see disease as an assault on the body from outside.

In the twentieth century, however, many such infections were controlled or conquered and – combined with public health measures and the reduction of infant mortality – this led to a huge increase in life expectancy. As a result, the main killers became heart disease and cancer, conditions usually associated with old age. But, whereas infections could clearly be understood as the outside world invading the body, heart disease and cancer looked more like the body's internal system going wrong by itself. We now know this is not quite true – both conditions can be caused by externalities – but it remains the case that these types of disorder, these dominant ways of dying, seem fundamentally different from infection.

Are such conditions discrete diseases in themselves or are they just the way in which nature imposes its system of programmed death? In fact, this question is raised even more acutely by the condition once simply known as dementia or senile dementia. Both terms, but particularly the latter, indicate that the decline of the intellect and memory was seen as a generalised deterioration rather than a specific pathology. Indeed, just as puberty might be seen as a natural accompaniment to growing up, so some degree of dementia might be seen as a normal accompaniment to growing old. In this light, dementia is not a disease at all, any more than puberty is. It lies, therefore, beyond the competence of doctors. This would have been a relief to the medical profession as it was – and remains – an incurable and all but untreatable condition.

But, in medicine, names matter. The dominant form of dementia had been identified as a distinct entity in the early twentieth century in Germany by Emil Kraepelin and its characteristic neuropathology was determined by his colleague Alois Alzheimer. But, curiously, the words 'Alzheimer's disease' were, at first, only uttered at the bedsides of forty-five- to sixty-five-year-olds who were said to be suffering from presenile dementia. The point seems to have been that to be demented after sixty-five was normal, to be demented before was abnormal – i.e. diseased. Thus to be old and sick was quite different from being young and sick. Irrational as this may now seem, it formed the basis of the scandalous lack of interest in geriatric medicine which was to persist into the 1970s and which still persists as an unspoken attitude in the minds of many doctors. Now, of course, Alzheimer's is the name given to a distinct set of symptoms manifested by any-body at any age. The dementia of the old has thus been brought within the realm of medicine merely by an act of naming. Very few now would argue that Alzheimer's is not a disease, though its exact physical basis remains elusive.

This trend towards the definition of all kinds of conditions as diseases rather than merely the inevitable results of the ageing process is partly economic. The wealthiest countries have, thanks to greater life expectancies and lower birth rates, ageing populations. And their elderly tend to be rich and able to pay for cures for their ailments. But more importantly – at least for my purposes – it is conceptual and directly linked to the revolution in thought about human ageing that culmi-nated in Tom Kirkwood's bath in 1977. If the body is not programmed to die, then there is no such thing as a dying process that is common to all and nor can ageing be regarded as a rite of passage like puberty. Rather, the body succumbs to a series of accidents against which it is increasingly unable to defend itself. These accidents may be individually classifiable as diseases. But there is no disease condition called old age, rather it is simply a collection of individual pathologies.

This dismissal of old age as a disease in itself lies at the heart of the immortalist programme. It also lay at the heart of the conflict that fired the delegates at Atlanta. Sherwin Nuland, the distinguished doctor who had written the profile of Aubrey de Grey in *Technology Review*, is the single most eloquent defender of the view that there is, indeed, such thing as old age. In his book *How We Die*, he wrote of the death of his old grandmother and the way 'cerebrovascular accident' (CVA) was written as the cause of death on her death certificate. For Nuland this was absurd – 'to tell me that the process I had been watching for eighteen years had ended in a named acute disease – well, it was illogical'.

He goes on: 'This is not simply a problem of semantics. The difference between CVA as a terminal event and CVA as a cause of death is the difference betweeen a worldview that recognizes the inexorable tide of natural history and a worldview that believes it is within the province of science to wrestle against those forces that stabilize our environment and our very civilization.'

Nuland is right to see this apparently obscure medical point as representing different worldviews. It is this insight that really led me to write this book. His is what the immortalists would call the 'deathist' position in a nutshell. It is 'natural' to die, it is part of the ancient order from which we sprang and which continues to sustain us.

Nuland says: 'Far from being irreplaceable, we should be replaced. Fantasies of staying the hand of mortality are incompatible with the best interests of our species and the continuity of mankind's progress.'

For Nuland, old age is a real and observable condition, not just a concatenation of accidents. Old people don't just look old outside, they look old inside. The brain and all the organs are stained yellowish-brown by a substance called lipofuscin, a product of the breakdown and absorption of damaged blood cells. (It is also the pigment that gives earwax its characteristic colour.) Age degrades every aspect of the body's appearance and function. Its effects, as evoked by Nuland, are total and catastrophic. It is, in his terms, simply absurd to try to reclassify this deluge of decay as a series of discrete conditions. It is what we always thought it was – old age.

You don't have to be a full-blooded immortalist to resist this idea. Kirkwood certainly does and Raymond Tallis, a prominent British geriatrician, has written of the way it 'is used as an excuse by ageist scoundrels wanting to deny health care to older people'. Nuland is certainly no scoundrel, but, historically, the medical professon has repeatedly used ageing as a way of evading actually having to deal with the problems of the old.

But, for the immortalists, it is absolutely essential to refute the Nuland position philosophically – we do not need to die for the good of the species – and medically – there is no one definable process of ageing, there are simply a number of fix-able events. The body, insists Aubrey de Grey, is a machine, it can be fixed; it is a form of mysticism to believe otherwise.

Almost by default, the immortalists are winning this argu-ment. The real reason they are doing so is neither philosophical nor medical but cultural. In *The Hour of Our Death*, Philippe Aries speaks of 'the invisible death' – the death, first identified by Geoffrey Gorer, that is utterly removed from society. It is removed by medical technology to the confines of the hospital, typically the intensive care ward. Gorer noted the way this made death as shameful a matter as pornography had once been. But Aries goes further.

> Technology erodes the domain of death until one has the illusion that death has been abolished. The area of the invisible death is also the area of the greatest belief in the power of technology and its ability to transform man and nature.
>
> Our modern mode of death was born and developed in places that gave birth to two beliefs: first, the belief in nature that seemed to eliminate death; next, the belief in a technology that would replace nature and eliminate death the more surely.

The cultural change brought about by modern technology thus prepares the way for the idea that death is, at heart, a technological matter.

Dead AND Alive

This idea has been further reinforced by one of the most familiar and yet one of the strangest medical developments of the modern era – the decidability of death. We now accept that doctors have the power to turn people on or off. Patients in 'persistent vegetative states' can be either kept alive or allowed to die. This seems unremarkable today, but it represents a transformation in our perception of death, a cultural change that, once again, strengthens the hand of the immortalists.

Death is, on the face of it, a black and white issue. There would seem to be no possibility of confusion. You cannot be partly dead. Losing a limb does not make part of you dead nor you as a whole more dead than you were before. This is because death means the end of 'you' as a functioning system, an identity. 'You are dead' is ungrammatical as there is no such thing as 'you' left that can be anything.

There have, however, always been some ambiguities. People have returned from what appeared to be death. Sometimes the apparently dead were left in special rooms before burial to ensure that they were, indeed, dead. And in Petro Voodooism in Haiti, the creation of zombies involves the use of – as the ethnologist Wade Davis discovered – tetrodotoxin, puffer fish poison, to induce a death-like state from which the victim could be brought back to life. Both examples seemed to imply a liminal state between death and life.

To the contemporary mind, these were simply errors. Anybody recovering before burial had simply been wrongly

diagnosed – either because of the primitive technology of the
time or because the definition of death as the cessation of the
heartbeat was simply inadequate. In Haiti, the apparent death
was induced pharmaceutically and was used as an assertion
of priestly power over life and death.

Yet contemporary medicine has not restored the absolute-
ness of death. Rather, it has massively increased our
uncertainties, expanded the liminal field. It did so by addressing the problem of definition. The traditional diagnosis of
death depended on the cessation of heartbeat and respiration. The doctor would feel for a pulse and/or place a mirror
over the mouth and nose. If it misted, there was breath and,
therefore, life.

There were always problems with this. Some people did
come back to life. If, at apparent death, the bodies were rapidly cooled, as a result, say, of falling into cold water, then
they could be brought back to life with no apparent damage
for up to an hour or more afterwards. It was thus always
clear that there was no absolute connection between death
and the usual indicators of lack of pulse and respiration –
rather these were just, usually, reliable signs.

The usual indicators were made even less reliable by the
development of resuscitation and life-support techniques.
Hearts could be restarted, breathing re-established.
Furthermore, transplant technology required that these be
done in order to preserve potentially usable organs in patients
whose brains were beyond hope of recovery. Brain death is
the way we have solved the resulting problems. Called 'irreversible coma', it was first advocated as a formal definition of
death in 1968 by a committee of Harvard Medical School
and was legally adopted a few years later. Now we routinely
accept that the death of a person's brain means the death of
that person, whatever the condition of the rest of his body.
This is still not completely clear-cut as we often do not know

if a coma is irreversible. People have recovered from apparent brain death. But, in terms of what we know, it is a more reliable indicator than the cessation of pulse or breathing.

The very act of redefinition is what counts. Medical knowledge and technology have created a new realm of liminality. A person who looks well, whose entire body except for his brain is functioning normally, can now be called dead. But he is only called dead because we can't fix his brain. Surely, therefore, he is only relatively dead. In fact, he is only called dead because of the limitations of our medical knowledge. In the future new procedures – nanotechnology, for example – may be able to rebuild his brain, restoring his memories and identity from the damaged molecules. The very fact that we have redefined death once must mean we can do it again. Death has been relativised.

The creation of a new realm – routinely seen in intensive care units – somewhere between life and death, has opened our minds to the possibility that our end is not quite so easily defined as we may have thought. It has opened our minds to the idea of technology somehow cradling us, carrying us safely through this last rite of passage or, indeed, abolishing the rite entirely. From Darwin to the idea of 'clinical' death, the direction is plain. We can first understand and then control what we had once taken to be our ultimate and inevitable destiny.

This idea gives me a feeling of vertigo. I shall now try to explain why.

3

The Mirror of Death

About Me (1)

'Death', wrote the Mexican poet Octavio Paz, 'is a mirror which reflects the vain gesticulations of the living.'

It is impossible to discuss or contemplate death without discussing and contemplating oneself. So here goes.

Immanuel Kant said we do not attain maturity until we are forty. Marcus Aurelius said that a man of forty had seen all there was to see. To the Enlightenment philosopher, life offered a virtual eternity of possible thoughts and ideas, of progress. To the stoical Roman Emperor, it only offered more of the same; you could watch the world for 10,000 years, it would still look much as it did after forty.

I have always, I know, lived on borrowed time. I was not a healthy child, multiply allergic, subject to every passing infection and frequently suffering from very serious asthma. Modern medicine in the form of violent physiotherapy, oxygen tents, adrenalin injections, steroids and an impressive number of ever-more exotic drugs kept me alive. In any other age I would not have survived. This is not so unusual. In any other age most people would not have survived. Life expectancies were much lower before the twentieth century came along with its antibiotics, sanitation and control of infant mortality. In that context, almost the entire contemporary population lives on borrowed time, time borrowed from the weapons, bureaucracies, sewers, architecture, agriculture, education and, latterly, health care provided by civilisation. Yet, still, I am aware of the artificiality of the continued existence of me in particular, aware that my debt to God has been deferred.

And now my time is doubly mortgaged. Both my parents died in their fifties, the same, in Aurelian terms, superfluous decade that I currently inhabit. If I am to consider my position with regard to matters of life and death, then I had better get on with it.

I did not see my father's corpse, though I saw my mother's and, with a brief shudder, I removed the watch from my father-in-law's dead wrist. There is an exact moment which explains both the first fact and the second, though it has nothing to do with the third. I shall, however, return to the shudder.

That moment was early in the morning in January. I was thirteen. I had woken to see my cousin Barrie's face, a pale oval floating in the half darkness. He was lying on the other bed, watching me. I asked him why he was there. He shouldn't have been, I remembered him leaving with his parents the night before. The exact choreography of that night's events still remains unclear to me. I know that doctors came and went, as doctors do.

I can't remember what Barrie said, but he walked with me down the corridor from my bedroom. He had placed himself between me and the door of my parents' room. I moved to go in there, but, just with pressure from his shoulder, he stopped me. Nothing was said but I did notice that the movement of his shoulder was slightly hurried. About five minutes later, I discovered my father had died and his corpse was in that room, hence the urgency. *He must not see*. I never did see the body.

Some years later, my mother died in a nursing home. I arrived with my brother. They had not told us she had just died. When they did, my brother flung some flowers to the floor. We were asked if we wished to see the body. My brother said no but I said yes. She was lying propped, for some reason, at an angle of about thirty degrees, her mouth wide open and her head flung back. She looked somehow stretched, as if she was trying to bite at something above her that she could not quite reach. My first instinct had been the same as my brother's, a squeamish impulse not to look. But, when asked, I had remembered the pressure of Barrie's shoulder and I felt I wanted to correct something, an omission. *This time I must see*. I said to my brother that she looked beautiful, but only to console him. In truth, she looked terrible, frightening.

As a child, I had – like, I am sure, most children – developed a fear of death that seemed to accompany me everywhere, sometimes like a friend. It was a secret, I could not divulge it to anybody, least of all my parents. Nobody ever talked about it so I thought I must be the only one with this fear. When I was eleven, this conspiracy became obvious and all but intolerable. During the Cuban Missile Crisis, we carried on living as normal and *nobody said anything*. Only I seemed to be thinking about the horrible death that was about to fall from the air. Clearly, given their apparent complacency, adults could not be suffering from the same fears. I assumed they must know something I didn't and would, therefore, regard my fears as ridiculous. Or they just expected the worst and thought it best to say nothing. *He must not know*.

Probably what they knew was religion. I went to church quite regularly with my father but the idea of Christian immortality did not penetrate my private world, though the idea of immortality itself certainly did. I quietly developed an entirely illogical theology of my own. I can't remember it in detail, but I know I thought there was a possibility that I would live forever if I was the Messiah. This made no sense in terms of what I had been taught, since, if there was such a thing as a Christian Messiah, then surely everybody would live forever.

I never really lost my secret belief in some kind of immortality. It is still here within me, though now 'belief' would be much too strong a word. The greatest challenge it faced in the intervening years was not loss of faith, but anaesthesia. I have had two trivial operations involving a general anaesthetic. In both cases, I was struck by the totality of the oblivion. Ordinary sleep – for me, at least – could not compare with this casual chemical elimination of my self. It does so much more than provide the premonitory 'temporary extinction' of which David Hume writes in his discussion of immortality. Under anaesthesia, the instants of going under and waking up were absolutely contiguous with no dreams and no moments of wakefulness to assure me that all was not lost. In the space in between, all was lost. I did not exist, just as, in the past, I did not exist and, in the future, I shall not exist. A belief in immortality that is inspired solely by incredulity at the possibility of non-existence of the self and its world must be shaken by such experiences.

Throughout my childhood, there was a giant figure watching me from the horizon, perhaps a couple of miles away at the low summit of some moorland that rose from the end of the lane where we lived. It was always there until, one day, it wasn't. Watched by this giant that nobody else could see – well, perhaps they could, typically I never mentioned it – and lost in my private theology, I acquired my lifelong conviction that the world was not as anybody else said it was. Or possibly they were all lying about what it was like. *He must not see and he must not know*. Either way, it was best to keep myself to myself.

This absolute conviction that adult accounts of the nature of the world were absolutely wrong has stayed with me. I simply cannot believe the world is as we are told it is. There is either something missing or something hidden behind the veil of ordinary reality. I will be obliged to confront this further in my later chapters on religion and spiritualism.

I did not see much of my cousin Barrie after that January morning when I saw his face, a pale oval floating in the half darkness. He wandered in and out of my life occasionally. But, eventually, all contact ended. Then, one day, a man I did not know phoned. He was an academic, a colleague of Barrie's. He was ringing to tell me Barrie had died. In his last illness, he had said specifically he wanted none of his family involved. His funeral had already taken place.

Years before, Barrie, a philosopher, had told me that if he ever produced his great work, it would be prefaced by Wallace Stevens's poem 'The Idea of Order at Key West'. I understood why. But the man who called said he had specified another poem to be read at his funeral – William Wordsworth's sonnet 'The World is Too Much With Us, Late and Soon'. I understood why again. They are, in some sense, the same poem.

Sylvia Anthony, in her book *The Discovery of Death in Childhood and After*, said that it is only 'above the age of seven do we find definition of *dead* as the negation of *living*'. Before that, death is seen as a condition within life so that, to the child, people can die and then come back to life. This is understandable: how would it be possible for anybody, child or adult, to conceive of a condition outside of life? As

Wittgenstein pointed out, death is not an event in life, we do not live through death. The logic of the child, therefore, is sound enough, based as it is on a disbelief in the possibility of a state beyond the knowledge of the person in that state. I am sure, in the contemporary world, that children are encouraged in their conviction that death is, somehow, inside life by films in which an actor can die in one and live again in another. My private theology does not seem so unusual, it is merely another example of the child seeing the problems with adult language, problems that society requires us to forget.

Anthony's book argues that there is a parallel between the logic of the child confronted by death and that of 'early man'. She points out that certain themes are common to all cultures. 'Phenomena which induce, in men of widely separated cultures, reasoning leading to similar conclusions are: the body perceived as separable from the soul, the world independent of the self, fate inexorable, time which goes only one way for man, and surely life under threat of death.'

'It is now our aim', she goes on, 'to show that the young child, ignorant like early man of many facts known to modern adults, capable like early man of logical reasoning, and like him unwilling to accept separation and non-existence, dissolution and decay, is led by the same phenomena as they to similar conclusions.'

The idea that modern adults know something which saves them from the delusions of early man is nonsense. But Anthony's point that there is a common matrix of human responses to death is important. Specifically her first theme – 'the body perceived as separable from the soul' – seems to be at the heart of the matter, primarily because of my sense of what a corpse actually looks like, especially when it is the corpse of somebody I knew.

Both my father-in-law and my mother looked, in death, not as dead people but as things from which a person had departed. If so, then the corpse itself cannot be dead because it is simply an empty container. What is actually 'dead' in the strict sense of 'gone forever' is the combination of the body with whatever has departed, a complete system. Yet the application of the word 'dead' to a corpse still seems obvious. Barmen often refer to empty glasses as 'dead', they are empty containers. But, if the drink has gone from the glass, what has gone from the corpse?

Earlier, I naturally used the word 'it' to denote my father's corpse, meaning, of course, that it was not 'him'. So this astonishing transition from a 'him' to an 'it' is death.

'My employment', says John Death in T.F. Powys's novel *Unclay*, 'is a simple one – I change one thing into another.'

The title of that novel denotes the process. The person is 'unclayed', removed from the clay of earth. But what actually happens in this change? The overwhelming feeling – not just for the 'early man' or the child but for anybody – is that something, if not somebody, has left this 'it' behind.

This sense of something leaving the body is reflected in the language. We talk of people who have 'departed this life', 'passed on', 'passed away', 'gone to a better place' and so on. Or we talk of human life as a process of passing through this world – 'passing through nature to eternity', says Gertrude in *Hamlet* – as if there were exits to elsewhere both before and after.

Even language which sounds neutral betrays our difficulty with the conception of death. 'He died' is a strange construction because 'he' did nothing of the sort. 'He' didn't die, he stopped being. 'Death happened to him' would be more accurate. That sort of construction makes sense of our attempts to personify death – as, for example, the Grim Reaper – because they make clear that death seems to attack us from the outside and that we are powerless to resist.

Of course, all the mystery can be stripped out of this with

one image – that of the machine. If a machine stops working, the mechanic doesn't think something has departed, he just thinks it has broken. A blocked fuel line will stop a car, turning it from a means of transport into a useless pile of metal. Similarly a blocked artery can turn a person into a corpse. Nothing has departed. All that has happened is that the system has ceased to support the activity for which it was designed. The activity of the system of the body is life, an activity that, in humans, includes the sub-activity we call self-consciousness.

This is true enough, but two points still nag at me. First, a person would only appear to be an activity to the driest of analytical philosophers. Machines are highly competent, but they have yet to attain, among other things, personal identity. Secondly, the car can be fixed by unblocking the fuel line, the person can't be fixed unless we unblock the artery very quickly. Cars could, in fact, be made immortal simply by continuously renewing their parts. That is, of course, what scientists are now planning to do to humans.

Discussions about what happens at death are not trivial word games. Talking about death is a routine social quandary. How do you speak to somebody who knows they are dying? Mostly, people avoid the issue because there is no issue. Just as we do not live through death, so there is no subject matter to be found in the condition of being dead. And yet this can be consoling. Once I was sitting by the hospital bed of my severely handicapped niece, making small talk because the next day she was to have a huge operation that might kill her. She was eleven. She condescendingly played the silly game of our small talk for a while, but when her doctor arrived she looked him in the eye and asked, 'Will I die?' 'You might,' he replied and her body seemed to relax.

What she thought at that moment I do not know, but I do know that the child who thinks death must be a condition within life is correctly seeing through the frailty of our language and, therefore, ourselves when it comes to death. More importantly, seeing death as a condition in life must mean that the child sees people as immortal. It is, in some way, *natural* to believe in immortality because the alternative belief – in our own or somebody else's complete cessation – simply cannot be entertained.

The Shudder

I could not stop myself shuddering when I removed the watch from my father-in-law's wrist. I would not have shuddered on contact with the dead flesh of an animal. Indeed, I daily consume the stuff. I don't even shudder on contact with living human flesh. But I don't eat humans and I do shudder on contact with their dead flesh.

This is the physical response to the imaginative conviction that something has departed this particular meat, something more significant than whatever has departed animal meat. It is the same response that led the Romans to fear corpses and to banish the tombs of the dead to the sides of the roads outside their towns. And, paradoxically, it is the same response that led most Christians – at least from the sixth century onwards – to hold on to their dead by burying them in the town, around or inside churches or, ideally, close to the bodies of the sainted martyrs. Banishing the corpse or holding on to it are both ways of saying the same thing: this is not ordinary meat, there is something special about it.

Corpses, one way or another, are awkward things, they cause an itch in the mind that can never be scratched. People want to say something about them or even to them, but they cannot find the words. Corpses have this power, a kind of authority. We know in our heads that they are only meat to be burned, buried or cut up. A degree of reverence might be fitting, nothing much. But, in our hearts, we know it is significant meat.

Even atheist, communist regimes succumb to the metaphysics of significant meat. Lenin's body was preserved in the Kremlin. It was against his own wishes, he despised such evidence of religiosity. But Stalin, his successor, understood religion and had the body embalmed to be venerated by the masses. They weren't supposed to feel such things on the way to communism's Utopia, but Stalin knew they would. This matter is sacred. It is not just matter, it is a sign of something else, of something beyond mere flesh. The shudder I felt at the touch of my father-in-law's dead flesh was religion.

When I visited Alcor in Scottsdale, Arizona, they took me into the room where they keep the frozen whole bodies or heads of their customers. Alcor is the leading company in cryonics, the practice of freezing dead people in the hope that they can be brought back to life in the future when technology allows. The big stainless steel flasks, Dewars, in which the customers are kept are never opened, so there was nothing especially alarming to be seen. The Dewars contain heads and whole bodies, the latter stored upside down to minimise the risk of brain damage in case of a coolant leak. I immediately found myself visualising the heads and the upside down bodies behind the opaque steel walls. I faint occasionally and I was beginning to feel light-headed. I edged out of the room and quickly recovered. In fact, this could have been caused by an excessive sensitivity to the coolant vapours in the room, some nitrogen continually boils off the tops of the Dewars. But, even if it was, my dizziness swirled around the imagined and terrible spectacle of those deep-frozen corpses standing on their heads. It was another shudder, but now with the added frisson that, in the eyes of Alcor and in some way beyond the reach of current medicine, these were not corpses at all but sleeping people.

The ambiguous matter of human meat has become a major cultural motif in recent years. This is, I think, because of the phenomenon – the denial of death and the suppression of outward signs of its occurrence – noted by Geoffrey Gorer in 1965 and Philippe Aries in 1977. This phenomenon was by no means universal in all its details; indeed, Gorer's view was that it was particularly English and Aries noted the American passion for embalming as opposed to the English enthusiasm for cremation. From the perspective of the sixties and seventies – things are slightly different now – it was universally true in the developed world that the process of dying, death itself and the grieving aftermath had been removed from common sight. Corpses didn't litter the streets, as they once did, nor did bones project from mass grave pits. When people became ill, they were admitted to hospital. If nothing could be done, they either died there or in some nursing home or hospice, only occasionally returning home. They were, therefore, quite likely to die among strangers and, if in intensive care, in a drugged haze, their bodies invaded by tubes as if being cyborged in preparation for the journey to the beyond.

Because people are getting much older thanks to medicine, many of them are in some sort of care long before they die. This isolation among strangers tightens a vicious circle identified by the German sociologist Norbert Elias: 'The fact that . . . the early isolation of the dying occurs with particular frequency in the more advanced societies is one of the weaknesses of these societies. It bears witness to the difficulties that many people have of identifying with the ageing and the dying.'

This concealment is further enforced by denial. Denial is reinforced by the administratively convenient convention of lying to the patient. It was seen as easier for relatives and it was certainly much easier for doctors and nurses if the patient was not actually told he was dying. Aries rightly sees this as a fundamental transformation in human affairs. The good death of the past was one in which the patient had complete knowledge and could prepare himself. Indeed, the unexpected death was regarded as a terrible curse, something to be feared and, if possible, avoided. Now the good death is the sudden death or the ignorant death and relatives are frequently consoled with words like 'He would have felt nothing' or 'He would have known nothing about it.'

'And everyone becomes an accomplice', writes Aries, 'to a lie born of this moment which later grows to such proportions that death is driven into secrecy. The dying person and those around him continue to play a comedy in which "nothing has changed", "life goes on as usual", and "anything is still possible".'

Gorer was equally appalled by this development, yet his emphasis is different in a curious way. He was drawn into lying to his brother Peter. Peter had terminal cancer but, somehow, everybody had agreed it would better if he wasn't told. Gorer acquiesces but feels intellectual rather than spiritual guilt: 'We shared a respect for the values of scientific knowledge which I felt were being transgressed.'

But perhaps the most extraordinary sign of this deep change in attitudes towards the dying came from the Catholic Church's Second Vatican Council (Vatican II) which lasted from 1962 to 1965. This is well known as the great liberalising moment of the Church, the moment when the papacy turned to face contemporary reality. But, on the matter of death, it did something rather different. The sacrament of Extreme Unction was renamed 'the anointing of the sick'. The priest arriving to deliver the 'last rites' to a person fully aware of their approaching death had become a thing of the past. The sacrament, as Aries remarks, had been detached from death.

In an essay entitled 'The Pornography of Death' in 1955,

Gorer had first drawn attention to this denial, removal and suppression of death and compared it to the Victorian suppression of sexuality. He writes: 'There seem to be a number of parallels between the fantasies which titillate our curiosity about the mystery of sex, and those which titillate our curiosity about the mystery of death.'

Exposing death, in other words, had become as taboo, as disgraceful, as exposing sex had once been and 'The natural processes of corruption and decay have become disgusting, as disgusting as the natural processes of birth and copulation were a century ago.' This is the crucial point that led directly to the renewed fascination with these processes over the last decade or so. For, of course, making death taboo endows it with the imaginative energy that sex once had.

And so in 1991 Damien Hirst exhibited his shark floating in a tank of formaldehyde with the title *The Physical Impossibility of Death in the Mind of Someone Living*. In the same year Marc Quinn exhibited his sculpture *Self*, a self-portrait of the artist made out of eight pints of his frozen blood. From the mid-nineties onwards Gunther von Hagens's Body Worlds exhibitions were seen by millions around the world. They consisted of plastically preserved corpses in grotesque and horrific poses. In 1999 David O. Russell's film *Three Kings* about the aftermath of the first Gulf War made a special point of showing, via animation, the internal effects of a bullet striking a body. The US TV series *Six Feet Under* about a family undertaking business in Los Angeles began in 2001. Meanwhile, the British journalist John Diamond outlined, in newspaper columns, on television and in a book, his slow death from throat cancer between 1997 and 2001. A society could only have found such an account remarkable if it had previously been in the habit of averting its eyes from the harsh reality of dying.

All of these works self-consciously exploited the death and

decay taboo. *Six Feet Under*, in particular, goes into immense detail about the process of retrieving, embalming and cosmetically enhancing corpses. We learn, if we did not know before, that corpses get erections – so-called 'Angel Lust' – that escaping air makes them emit horrible noises and that they frequently defecate. We also learn of the extraordinary efforts made by American undertakers to conceal the deeply unattractive effects of death on the human body. The use of two tins of cat food to prop up a porn star's epic breasts sticks in the mind.

The breaching of the sexual taboo having been exhausted as a goad to the contemporary imagination and, in any case, sex of every variety having become banal and mainstream, death has risen up to take its place. This meat, say these works, is *all* that you are. They can say this because the suppression of death had worked. People had forgotten about mere death. Diamond's cancer story was, in this context, an exposé.

Two very successful books also captured this motif of the rediscovery of the meat. In *Stiff: The Curious Lives of Human Cadavers*, published in 2003, the American journalist Mary Roach jauntily confronts meat anxiety by recounting what happens to corpses. They are used for medical research, for teaching, for testing car safety, for military research, for investigating plane crashes and so on. The joke running through the book is the way Roach writes about the 'activities' of the corpses. She treats them as if they were like living people busily engaged in doing something useful, as if they had an afterlife. But her imagination is strictly secular and the message of the book is that we should neither be squeamish nor pious about our dead bodies, rather we should be pleased they can be put to some use.

But, of course, her book was a success – it was a *New York Times* bestseller – precisely because most people have not yet accepted her matter-of-fact, serenely humanist approach. If they had, her tales of post-mortem adventures would seem unremarkable.

It is, however, the formidable *How We Die: Reflections on Life's Final Chapter* by Sherwin B. Nuland, published in 1993, that most honestly confronts the new way of dying, identified by Aries and Gorer, and most persuasively advocates a new secular engagement with the process. In addition, as I have said, Nuland is opposed to one of the key beliefs of the new longevity movement – that we are killed by disease, not by old age.

On the matter of the meat, Nuland, a doctor, is unrelenting. Almost without exception, humans do not die well: 'The quest to achieve true dignity fails when our bodies fail. Occasionally – very occasionally – unique circumstances of death will be granted to someone with a unique personality, and that lucky combination will make it happen, but such a confluence of fortune is uncommon, and, in any case, not to be expected by any but a very few people.'

Typically, our deaths, even in hospital, are miserable, fluid-soaked messes and/or harrowing disintegrations of the personality. As a result: 'The good death has increasingly become a myth. Actually, it has always been for the most part a myth, but never nearly as much as today. The chief ingredient of the myth is the longed-for ideal of "death with dignity".'

In saying that old age does, indeed, kill people, Nuland is drawing attention to the totality of the failure that is death: 'The sequence of events by which tissue and organs gradually yield up their vital forces in the hours before and after . . . death are the true biological mechanisms of dying.'

Nuland is taking the Aries–Gorer evocation of a ritualised, secular death one step further. He is saying that, if we are to come to terms with death, it is precisely *this*, this dignity-free implosion of our bodies that we must confront.

But such a confrontation with harsh reality also confronts the idea of significant meat and thus threatens the ritualised basis of the old observance of death. If, at death, we become the corrupted mess that Nuland describes, should we really be expected to honour these hideous remains? Should we pretend they have anything to do with the person they once embodied? I have frequently heard of relatives of Alzheimer's patients counselled not to regard the deranged mass of incoherent responses they see before them as the person they once knew. This is equivalent to saying they died before the onset of the later stages of the disease. It is undoubtedly humane, well-meant, but it has the effect of saying this body has lost all relevance. It is an empty vessel. Should we hold funerals for people while they are still alive?

Aries discusses the macabre art of the medieval period, the sudden appearance of gruesome imagery that, like the work of Hirst or Quinn, drew attention to our bodily reality. In the eleventh century Odilon of Cluny spoke of 'that which is hidden in the nostrils, in the throat, in the bowels: filth everywhere'. Later this horror became a genre in the visual arts. Conventionally such art is seen as a warning about impending death and judgement, a straightforward memento mori. But, to Aries, they represent the first signs of secularisation because they show a sudden love for materiality, for the things of this world. He writes: 'The images of death and decomposition do not signify fear of death or the beyond . . . They are the sign of a passionate love for this world and a painful awareness of the failure to which each human life is condemned.'

Similarly, the macabre fascinations of our day arise from dismay and disgust at the eclipsing of our material existence. It is a transgression that breaks through the denial of death just as an earlier transgression had broken through the denial of sex. But, having liberated sex, you can at least have sex; it is not clear what can be done once death has been set free.

The prospect of medical immortality thus looms before us at a time when our understanding – both intellectual and intuitive – of what death is, what it means and how we should react to it is in transition. Like a funeral guest confronted with the bereaved, we do not know what to say.

Guilt

'Tell me how you die,' wrote Octavio Paz, 'and I will tell you who you are.'

This is an incredible claim. I could die by being shot in the back of the head and my death would be indistinguishable from that of millions of others who have been shot in the back of the head. And yet, deep within us, there remains the perhaps irrational conviction that death is the ultimate mirror, it shows us who we are.

'I had become', wrote St Augustine when recalling the death of a close friend, 'a question to myself.'

It is the death of the other that provokes the question, who am I? But the question is asked because the death of the other implies the death of oneself. An immortal could defer the answer indefinitely. But, for a mortal, the question must be urgent. It demands an end, a final answer, therefore it demands a death. Death, in this version, becomes the final summation, the final saying of oneself. Life is a story that has an end. Without death, there is the possibility, therefore, that one's story could never be told. We would be left with no self, just an endless state of becoming.

The problem of the story of the self is a serious one for the boosters of medical immortality. Even though we are still likely to die eventually, we would have difficulties in seeing ourselves as a continuous story. Assume, for the purposes of argument, that the scientists have managed to make the brain more or less as immortal as the rest of the body. This is, of course, their central problem, but, as we shall see later, there are possible solutions. The brain accumulates memories. We do not know how it does this but we do know that the mechanism is very rapid. If you tell me your name, I remember it at once. We also know that short-term memories like that are, selectively, laid down as long-term memories. This requires space rather than speed. The unit of memory that carries your name must be very small – most likely a molecule – because, as well as your name, I have millions of other memories. Furthermore, a disconnected heap of memories would be useless, so I must also have complex connections between these memories that make them into narratives, associative patterns. And all of these must be stored inside the space of my skull.

It is obvious to me, an ageing boomer, that this storage/pattern-making system has limits. In my twenties I know I used to carry dozens of phone numbers in my head, now I have to look up all but a very few. I like to think – I hope – that this is because my brain is so full rather than because it is degenerating. But, even if it is because it is degenerating, it is clear that there must be a storage capacity problem for the brain as its temporal mileage accumulates.

If this is so, then the thousand-year-old is going to have a very serious problem. What, exactly, is he going to remember – the last hundred years with perhaps a few fragments from the previous nine hundred? Leon Kass has used this point to argue that the pursuit of medical immortality is futile. It would turn me into not an immortal self, but rather a series of mortal selves, a continuously dying population that only looked like one person. If I forget everything that happened to me between, say, the ages of hundred and two hundred, it must be true to say that that self has died.

Being told at a thousand about what we had done in those years would be rather like being told, as one occasionally is, that one has been reincarnated many times but one does not know it. What difference does it make? However many times I am reincarnated, my life, to me, will remain only this passage from my birthday to my deathday. So, to the thousand-year-old, his life will remain only the last century at best.

Of course, the same is true now with regard to much of our childhood self. I don't think I remember anything very much until I was about three when I believe I overheard my mother complaining about me to my father – 'He never stops talking!' But I have no idea why I think I was three as opposed to any other age. And, if I was so talkative, surely I was mentally competent enough to be laying down lasting memories. I could, of course, reconstruct much of my childhood self from other memory fragments, from talking to my brother or from physical objects – most obviously photographs – from the time. But much of this would probably be inaccurate as, usually, when I check my detailed memories of the past against other people's, they conflict.

The central point is that any such reconstruction will remain just that, a reconstruction or possibly a re-collection. It will not be a full-blooded memory. It would be akin to remembering what somebody looks like – big nose, dark hair, whatever – as a kind of police photofit rather than as the real image of the person called to mind, a re-collection. Vladimir Nabokov once said that this 'real image' remembering of a dead loved one was one of the greatest feats of which the human imagination is capable. At least I think he did. I can't remember where he said it. Anyway, I feel he is right and I can still 'see' rather than just re-collect my father. It is a great feat because it feels like a resurrection.

Perhaps this is evidence against Kass. The impact of the

event of my father's death might have been such that, aged a thousand, I shall still be able to 'see' his face, still be able, to that extent, to claim I am the same person I was at thirteen. Yet one feels that Kass must be right in the sense that, even if I could do that, most of the emotional and contextual attachments, most of the meaning of the image, would have long since vanished. I would be left with an odd mental trick that seemed to have no significance.

The tougher, philosophical argument against Kass has been formulated by John Harris, a philosopher at Manchester. Even if we accept, says Harris, that we will forget whole periods of our lives, this is not necessarily a catastrophe. Say we divide our lives up into periods *a*, *b* and *c*. Memory loss may mean that in period *c*, we cannot remember period *a*, but we can remember period *b*. Period *b*, meanwhile, will be a period in which we remember *a*. There will thus be a real continuity. In period *c* we may not remember period *a* directly but we will remember a period when we did. We shall have memories of memories. Clearly, over a thousand years there will be many more than just three such periods, but the point will still hold.

'I will not have to fear extinction if I am made immortal,' says Harris, 'though what I will fear is something different. I will fear losing memories – psychological continuity. Well, I have a real sense of psychological continuity with myself at three, though I can't remember what it was like. The memories I think I have are probably memories of memories, supplemented by externals – photograph albums, diaries, by memoirs, things you don't remember yourself. So there is a continuity even when memory fails.'

The, as it were, Nabokovian objection to this would be that memories of memories are just re-collections, rather than the emotion-saturated acts of recall. One would be seeing oneself as vividly as, say, watching a film of what one did.

One would not be reliving the experience. But Harris is only saying there will be *some* continuity and that should be enough to justify living rather than being dead.

Another anti-immortality argument, which Kass also advocates but which is most famously advanced by Francis Fukuyama, springs from a specific conception of human nature. This goes back to the Greek idea that humans are the only mortal things. Nature does not die, gods do not die and animals are only aspects of a species, not individuals, therefore they do not die. The slightly more modern version of this would be to say that only we *know* we are going to die, which is why Yeats can say, 'Man has created death.' If this is the case then dying and knowing we are going to die must be one of – if not the primary – the essential qualities of humanity. If we stop ourselves dying, therefore, we become post-human, some other kind of entity.

To respond by saying 'So what?, it will be better to be an entity that doesn't die,' is to miss the deeper point. The problem hinges on evaluative words like 'better'. Such words only make sense within narrow limits. This is why it has always sounded so strange to me when people speak, as they so often do these days, of 'enhancing' or 'improving' the human species. We can't know what an enhancement of the human would be because we only have the human to go on. You can't say, for example, that the space shuttle is an enhancement of a kettle. It is simply a different thing and, if a kettle thinks it would like to improve itself by becoming a shuttle, then it is making an obvious mistake. It can't still be its kettle self while being a spacecraft self. What it really means is that it would like to stop being a kettle. There is nothing intrinsically progressive in such an aspiration.

Of course, we can see things wrong with human beings, but the things that are wrong in one context are right in others. Bill Gates's surplus energy makes him difficult to talk to; he rocks back and forth all the time. On the other hand, it probably makes him a good boss of a big company. Furthermore, all attempts to change human nature for the better – the best example being communism – have sunk in a sea of blood. In practice, all enhancement ever means is the amplification of one aspect of our humanity. Since we know all such aspects – intelligence, skill, imagination, whatever – can never have only desirable outcomes, then we must know that such a change is as likely to have many bad effects as good ones. If we make ourselves 'post-human' by making ourselves immortal, then everything else, apart from our medical condition, will still be suffused with the residue of the human. From that perspective, it seems pretty likely that the first use of immortalising technology will be to produce new, improved soldiers. I don't think, when one of these guys puts a gun in your face, you would still argue that it is 'better' that he is immortal.

In fact, being a believer in betterment, that is probably not how Fukuyama would put it. But the general argument that to try to make us in- or post-human is either doomed or unwise is clear. Either it is conceptually incoherent and as likely to be as riven with error as any other human project or it will destroy human nature and thus the stability of the species.

The counter-argument is equally clear. Just because we don't understand all the consequences doesn't mean we shouldn't do something. Columbus did not anticipate *The Simpsons* and the invasion of Iraq when he set sail. He probably just had some vague, desirable goals – wealth, power, knowledge. Had he disliked *The Simpsons*, could that have been a good reason to stay in port? Hardly – not only because he had never seen the show, but also because it would seem to be an excessively fastidious view. But were his own aspirations good enough reason to leave? The answer is that leaving, striking out for distant places, moving on, seeking knowledge is what human beings have always done. It is as much a part of human nature as anything imagined by the anti-immortalist. And so, if it is human nature to transcend the human, then so be it. It is what we are, it is what we do. Freezing ourselves in our present human state would be worse than moving on.

Once we have moved on, our present feelings about death should, ideally, have been eliminated. Maybe. But what are these feelings? There is no one answer, of course, but guilt must be in there somewhere. The Shakespearean construction that we owe God a death means that, by being born, we plunge into debt. Or, to put it another way, to be born is to take a kind of liberty, to offend against our own non-existence.

'You are ceasing to be something which you would have done better never to have become,' were Schopenhauer's words to a dying man.

Death is, after all, the default condition of the universe. So far, it seems, only Earth sustains life, the rest is just dead matter. We think of death as a negative condition – not-life – but, to the cosmos, life is the negative condition – not-death. If we are to talk of nature, then, to a more or less unarguable approximation, it is completely dead.

This is not empty, metaphysical arm-waving. Feeling wrong in the world, an intruder, is not so much normal as universal. Nobody is ever completely at ease with themselves, it is yet another condition of being human. What precisely consti-tutes this ill-at-easeness was best put to me by the philosopher Roger Scruton:

'All existence in this world involves a struggle against others, overcoming of others to some extent and doing wrong to others and that is part of the contingencies of moral life. We always end up by the time we've won through to our freedom with an acquired burden of guilt, guilt towards parents, towards people who've loved you and cared for you . . . Not to have acquired that guilt is not to be free . . . There should be this residue of guilt that has to be worked through and overcome – largely through loving others and loving children especially as a cure for guilt. That puts you in the same position as your victims.'

'And, if you did away with the death which is the expiation of this guilt?' I asked him.

'I would have thought you would have a society of people with very much hardened hearts. People wouldn't need each other in the way that they do now. They'd all be sitting in their cubicles taking their pills. But, of course, they might make themselves invulnerable to disease but not to each other.'

Your death pays a debt, if not to God, then to your society. You must pay the price everybody else has paid. Death represents a completion, perhaps a perfection, of your existence. It turns your life into a story by providing the ending that ties all the loose ends together. This idea lies deep within people. It is a commonplace to hear people remark that the faces of corpses look 'at peace' or as if the deceased is simply sleeping. The dead person has found an answer to the question of his life and their serene appearance in death is evidence of the satisfaction this provides. In the United States, where the viewing of the embalmed corpse is a normal custom, this discovery of peace by the living in the dead has been extensively ritualised.

The completion of a story idea is also present in the popular myth that, at the moment of death, your entire life flashes before your eyes. Some who have been brought back from the brink of death actually report this occurrence, but its persistence in the culture is probably more to do with the way it fits into a religious tradition of which people remain dimly aware.

This tradition is that of the judgement of the life which takes place *at the moment of death*. The distinction I am stressing here is between the instantaneous judgement on death and the temporally distant judgement that occurs on the collective Day of Judgement. The vision of a final reckoning when the virtuous go to heaven and the wicked to hell is not, as many think, simply a changeless feature of Christianity. Initially, the assumption was that the dead were sleeping in the earth. When the time came, the virtuous were woken and taken to heaven and the wicked just left in the nothingness of death. This began to change in the Middle Ages. The theme of the Last Judgement itself began to appear in the eleventh century and went on to become a central theme of Renaissance art. Here the wicked were also woken and consigned to hell. But, still, there had been a period of sleep for all of the dead. Grand medieval tombs commonly have sculptures of the occupants in the repose of sleep, complete with a stone pillow.

In the seventeenth century, portrayals of death-bed scenes, which until then had simply shown family and friends around the bed, started depicting a new cast of characters – angels and demons – that were only visible to the dying person. What had happened was that the moment of judgement had been transferred from some distant time in the future to the moment of death. The angels and demons are fighting over the ultimate fate of this man. He will be judged 'in the twinkling of an eye'. The distant, collective courtroom of the Last Judgement has been replaced by the small, private hearing in the bedroom.

This seems to be, to the modern imagination, consoling. There is plenty of popular cultural evidence that instant judgement is preferable to a long wait. The film *Ghost* (Jerry Zucker 1990), for example, is based on the presumption that the bad are dragged straight to hell by grasping, ghostly shadows and the good, having been given a brief period to put things right, are drawn immediately up into a bright light in the sky. The period of putting things right is a therapeutic, rather than eschatological, version of the completion of the life story. In *Flatliners* (Joel Schumacher 1990), a group of young doctors decide to test the reality of life after death by rendering themselves 'clinically' dead and then bringing themselves back to life. What they encounter on the other side is a gothically dramatised therapy session in which they confront the unfinished business of their lives. The old drama of judgement is turned into the new drama of therapeutic atonement. The same theme is embodied slightly differently in the film and television convention of the conversation with the dead at the grave. This is when characters discuss their problems, usually with a dead wife, mother or father, by addressing their headstone. They look at this stone as if it were, indeed, a mirror.

There are several implications of this absolute contiguity of death and judgement – some of which I shall discuss later – but here the important point is that the act of dying becomes the final rounding off of the biography. There is no long wait, sleeping in the ground, for the story to be concluded; rather, it all happens at once. In our time this idea remains strong both in the myth of 'my life flashing before my eyes' and in the more organised mythology of the Near Death Experience (see Chapter Five). In NDEs people commonly report feeling themselves removed from their body and being drawn towards a bright light. There is often some kind of choice involved, again some assessment of the life is being made, often called the Life Review, though the horror of damnation has been banished from this version of the end.

Or, conceivably, this points to the possibility of being damned by *not* dying. If a life needs to be rounded off by a death, then evading death may be seen as a failure. That could be the consequence of making ourselves immortal at some point in the future. But there is a very vivid point in the past which provoked in many the guilt of not dying.

That point was at 8.15 a.m. on 6 August 1945, the moment at which the atom bomb exploded over Hiroshima. Tens of thousands died at once and many more later from injuries or radiation. Those that survived – known in Japanese as *hibakusha*, bomb-affected people – had endured an experience unprecedented in human history.

'The most striking psychological feature of this immediate experience,' writes Robert Jay Lifton, 'was the sense of a sudden and absolute shift from normal existence to an over-whelming encounter with death.'

In his book *Death in Life: Survivors of Hiroshima*, Lifton characterises the primary condition of the survivors as a complete failure to, in the cant phrase often used by television reporters, 'come to terms' with what has happened to them. They have found no peace with their fate. They feel guilty at having failed to die. The guilt is not rational. They did not drop the bomb. But it is real and, as Lifton has pointed out, they 'take on special burdens of responsibility and guilt for the over-all cosmic disruption, as well as for the "homeless dead" – those spirits which (according to folk cultures throughout the world) remain restless and dangerous through having died violently, unnaturally, and without proper ritual'.

There is such a thing as guilt at not dying. At Hiroshima it was born of military technology; it could equally well be born of medical.

A Bird Had Nested on His Breast

But the more usual punishment for living does not rely on your conscience; it depends on your body. The body signals the fall towards death in the most cruel and brutal manner.

From our twenties onwards we fall apart in increasingly humiliating ways until, finally, having been kept alive by modern medicine, we find ourselves bristling with tubes in intensive care or quietly rotting, amidst our coevals, in some nursing home or hospice. This process mocks all our ambitions and aspirations. Whatever we achieve, we will be slowly tortured by time until, finally, it releases us to return to the dust from which we came. A frequently used literary twist to this macabre joke is that even if we achieve immortality, old age still takes its revenge.

In one Greek myth, Eos, the goddess of the dawn, falls in love with the mortal Tithonus. She begs Zeus to make him immortal and her wish is granted. But she forgets to ask for his eternal youth. As a result, Tithonus cannot die, though he ages and withers, finally becoming a grasshopper and his voice could not be heard. Death, as Tennyson saw, would be a great blessing to Tithonus:

> *And after many a summer dies the swan.*
> *Me only cruel immortality*
> *Consumes.*

Similarly, the Cumean sybil, trapped forever in her bottle, is left with only one wish – 'I want', she says, 'to die.' To the immortal, mortality is the only aspiration left.

The trap of immortality is eternal old age and senility. In *Gulliver's Travels*, written in 1726 as Enlightenment rationality was beginning to take hold of the European mind, Jonathan Swift's hero encounters the Struldbruggs on the island of Luggnugg. Occasionally a Luggnugg child is born with a red circular spot over its left eyebrow. This is not an inherited condition, it occurs purely by chance. The spot grows larger and, when the child is twelve, turns green, then, at twenty-five, blue and, finally, at forty-five, black. The Struldbruggs go on to live forever. Gulliver, a reasonable eighteenth-century man, is enraptured: 'Happy nation where every Child has at least a Chance of being immortal! ... Exempt from the universal Calamity of Human Nature ... Without the Weight and Depression of Spirits caused by the continual Apprehension of Death.'

Gulliver imagines what he would do if he were immortal: 'I would first resolve by all Arts and Methods whatsoever to procure myself Riches: In pursuit of which, by Thrift and Management, I might reasonably expect in about two Hundred Years, to be the wealthiest Man in the Kingdom.'

He would form an academy of the immortals, rather like London's Royal Society. He says: 'What wonderful Discoveries should we make in Astronomy, by outliving and confirming our own Predictions; by observing the Progress and Return of Comets, with the Changes of Motion in the Sun, Moon and Stars.'

Gulliver is brought down to earth by the discovery that, like Tithonus, the Struldbruggs have been freed from death, but not from old age, that they 'pass a perpetual life under all the usual Disadvantages which old Age brings along with it'. Up to the age of thirty they generally live as other people, but then they descend into melancholy. At eighty 'they not only had all the Follies and Infirmities of other old Men, but many more which arose from the dreadful Prospect of never dying. They were not only opinionative, peevish, covetous, morose, vain, talkative; but incapable of Friendship and dead to all natural Affection ... At Ninety they lose their Teeth and Hair; they have at that age no Distinction of Taste, but eat and drink whatever they can get, without Relish or Appetite.'

Removing death as the inevitable outcome of bodily decay is a cruel and unusual punishment. There is consolation in this, as the persistence of this story through the centuries indicates. When young, we shudder at the condition of the old and think it would be better to be dead; when old, we know our infirmity will not last forever. Fear of death is eased by horror at the spectacle of old age.

But there is, perhaps, a still greater horror, a kind of appalling inflation of Marcus Aurelius's sense that the world has not enough in it to sustain our interest beyond the age of forty. In Jorge Luis Borges's short story 'The Immortal' a man goes off in search of 'the secret river which cleanses men of death'. He finds a river. There are people there, inert and apparently miserable. He engages one in conversation. These people are, indeed, the immortals. He asks this man what he knows of the *Odyssey*. 'Very little,' he replies, 'less than the poorest rhapsodist. It must be a thousand and one hundred years since I invented it.'

The man is Homer. The story goes on: 'Homer composed the *Odyssey*; if we postulate an infinite period of time, with infinite circumstances and changes, the impossible thing is not to compose the *Odyssey*, at least once.'

For the immortals in Borges's story all things happen to all men. This made them perfectly tolerant, but also indifferent. Nothing mattered because everything that could happen would happen. The immortals, as a result, can barely bring themselves to move: 'I remember one who I never saw stand up; a bird had nested on his breast.'

The problem of what to do with immortality or even with an extended life is profound and persistent in all discussions I have had on the subject. Life extension and immortality enthusiasts tend to be briskly optimistic.

'There will be a greater necessity for education and training,' says Aubrey de Grey, '. . . nobody with a good education gets bored, only those people who have never been given the skill to make a lot out of life.'

Nick Bostrom, an Oxford philosopher, speaks of enlarging the brain to cope with maintaining interest in almost limitlessly extended life, though, he adds, this might not be necessary for everybody: 'With immortality you would need to have your brain expand without limit . . . But, at the same time, a lot of people seem quite happy even though they don't change very much – they take a stroll in the park every morning, they have a nice cup of tea. It's not less pleasurable because you've done it every day.'

In contrast to this, the average person tends immediately to raise the problem of boredom, or even of weariness with a world that constantly seems to go wrong. Some change their minds when I point out that the new longevity would involve rejuvenation, restoring them to the age of about twenty-nine. I think the point here is that anybody over forty tends to think that all adventure, change, incident, happens when they are young. At some point – say, around thirty-five – this ends, to be replaced by routine and responsibility, a state of affairs that persists until the beginning of old age, at which point serious physical decline sets in. Thus immortality or extreme longevity to a forty-year-old may, at first, seem unattractive, but restoring him to twenty-nine would offer the prospect of a renewal of excitement. Nevertheless, the fact remains that most people are not enthused by the idea of going on forever. It may be, as de Grey and Bostrom both believe, that this lack of enthusiasm is a defensive ploy. People don't seriously think they can evade death and so they pretend they welcome it.

Maybe these immortality optimists are right. But the problem of boredom is profound and is not simply a case of not having enough to do. (I shall return to boredom in my final chapter.) The concept of death as the completion of a story is not just a way of viewing the whole of life but also a way of seeing life from moment to moment. For, in fact, we only seem to be able to understand our feelings at all when they are balanced against opposing feelings, as in a rounded-off story. So, when we feel happy, we feel it in contrast to being sad; when we feel at peace, we feel it in contrast to being anxious or insecure. We can't feel any good things unless we know they involve the absence of bad things.

'Why is there no lasting pleasure?' asked Ludwig Feuerbach. 'Because a continuing, an uninterrupted pleasure would no longer be experience and pleasure; pleasure is pleasure only because it passes away.'

It is, it seems, in the fleetingness of things that we experience the most intense pleasure and, indeed, sorrow. Flowers move us precisely because they bloom and die so rapidly. Imagine being shown a flower that was real but that had been engineered never to fade and die. Something, perhaps everything, would have been lost. Maybe we could learn to love it. But something very fundamental would have to be different about this love.

Borges's immortals are bored, not merely because there is nothing to do but because there is no point in doing anything. Given enough time, logically everything that can happen must happen, so why bother doing it now? The world has lost its savour, its excitement. The point is intensified by the fact that it is Homer that is the exemplar. The man and his work are the archetypes of artistic immortality. We can imagine future societies in which many things will be lost, but not Homer and not the *Odyssey*. And yet, take death away, and both become meaningless, futile. Death, therefore, grants purpose. What are we to do without it?

Love

Just about every scheme for life extension has demanded some restriction on sex. In the second and third centuries BC Chinese Taoists evolved a programme for attaining immortality that depended crucially on the avoidance of passion and sensuality in the pursuit of *wu wei* – 'effortless action'.

The early Taoist adepts considered the loss of *ching* – essence, but also sperm or menstrual fluid – as a threat to longevity. Yet they approved of sex. The compromise was a rite of intercourse involving *coitus reservatus*, the man did not ejaculate, though he would repeatedly be engaged with intercourse, ideally with girls aged between fourteen and nineteen. When, eventually, he had to orgasm, he had to clutch the urethra so that there was no ejaculation. We would now know he was diverting the semen to the bladder, but to the ancient Taoists he was conserving the *ching* in the body's 'lower field of cinnabar' where it would act as a rejuvenating substance.

The conviction that ejaculation involves more than just the loss of sperm is persistent. Balzac is supposed to have said 'there goes another novel' after orgasm. And the orgasm is, of course, often called 'the little death', perhaps because it is one of the few occasions when we experience the end of a process and a distinct mental transformation. In the twentieth century the Viennese physican Eugen Steinach evolved a surgical way of enforcing *coitus reservatus*. Effectively, this was a vasectomy. But Steinach thought the preservation of the fluid would rejuvenate his patients. The surgeon Serge Voronoff became convinced that, because the reproductive cells appeared to be better protected from ageing than the rest of the human body, they must contain an anti-ageing hormone. As we grow older, the amount of this hormone must decrease. Voronoff's solution was to take wedges of monkey testicle and insert them into a man's testicles. Obviously this resulted in rejection.

To both Steinach and Voronoff, sex and ageing and therefore death were linked as they had been for the Taoists. The thirteenth-century alchemist Roger Bacon endorsed this idea by suggesting the breath of young virgins as a source of rejuvenation for old men. This was not just young women, it was young *virgins*, indicating again the conviction that some vital force was lost in the act of sex. It is an idea that seems to have come from the Old Testament in which old King David lay with a beautiful maiden with whom he did not have sex. In our time Mahatma Gandhi would sleep between two young virgins, though, apparently, to test and prove his control of his libido.

Gandhi's technique points to another aspect of the connection between sex and death. Whereas these other devices were intended to prolong life here on earth by controlling sex, the more familiar idea is the control of sex in order to achieve immortality in heaven. Thus most of the major religions tend to promote, with different degrees of severity at different times, strict injunctions against promiscuity and equally strict endorsements of either marriage or celibacy. Particularly in the writings of St Paul, there seems to be something specifically wrong with sex which gets in the way of the process of salvation. Whether this amounts to a perversion of the teachings of Jesus or not is a matter of some dispute.

There is, in fact, no easy generalisation about religious attitudes towards sex beyond saying that it is taken seriously enough to be intimately involved with the issue of salvation or transcendence. It is also broadly possible to say that some restriction of sexual activity is, as with the Taoists and others, regarded as a good thing – though Paul did, in fact, suggest married couples should have a lot of sex, primarily to prevent any adulterous or homosexual activity.

Restriction of sex takes a slightly different form in the scheme for medical immortality that inspired this book. It does not discourage sex itself. But, if successful, it would require control of reproduction as a massive reduction of death rates would require an equally massive reduction of birth rates to prevent an uncontrollable growth in population. The usual solution offered to this problem involves making everybody that took longevity treatment sign an agreement not to have children. They could subsequently have children, but only if they then agreed to die. This is practical, but the idea has theological and mythological foundations that link it to sperm as the expendable essence of the self and undefiled virginity as the best, purest tribute to eternity. 'And in the cult of virginity', wrote the Spanish philosopher Miguel de Unamuno, 'may there not perhaps be a certain obscure idea that to perpetuate ourselves in others hinders our own personal perpetuation?'

Reproduction as a form of decay, a step towards dissolution, has roots in alchemy. Paracelsus, the sixteenth-century Swiss alchemist and physician, thought that all things 'naturally generated' arose from putrefraction. Thus sperm putrefied in the body of the woman to produce a child. 'For putrefaction', he wrote, 'is the chief degree and first step to generation . . .'

To reproduce is to decay or, in contemporary terms, to overpopulate. The idea of being forced to avoid this problem by restricting reproduction inspires interesting reactions. In Cambridge market, I offered a lady of around forty-five a Tune, actually a small, sweet, purple lozenge that 'helps you breathe more easily'. I was pretending it was an immortality pill. She was a stallholder, slim and fit looking but still dressed in far too young a style – denim miniskirt, wide hip-hugging belt, etc. She knew the pill was a fake, but became unusually involved in the idea. She said, as most people do, that she would not take it. But, I said, it will make you twenty-nine again. At once she said she would take it. But there is a catch, I said, you must agree not to have children. She had two daughters whom, plainly, she loved dearly. She looked bereft as if, for a moment, the choice was real. She would not under those circumstances take the pill. It would, in her imagination, be like wishing her daughters away.

The prospect of the death of the beloved other is what gives most people pause on the matter of immortality. Many say they are ready or happy to die, resigned to death. Few claim to be equally sanguine about the death of friends, children, spouses or parents. It does not seem so selfish, so small-minded, so ungenerous, to wish immortality on them. Indeed, it seems the obvious concomitant of love. 'The thirst of eternity', wrote Unamuno, 'is what is called love among men, and whosoever loves another wishes to eternalize himself in him. Nothing is real that is not eternal.'

Also at the final limit of our own life, we take consolation from the survival of others – not others in general but others in particular, those we have loved.

Philip Larkin, a secular man stricken by occasional stabs of religious longing, wrote a poem about a medieval tomb in Chichester Cathedral – that of Richard Fitzalan, Earl of Arundel, and Eleanor, his second wife. The sculpture of the couple, apparently asleep as was the custom at the time, shows them holding hands. This strikes Larkin with 'a sharp tender shock'. The sculpture, the poem concludes, has come 'to prove / Our almost instinct almost true: / What will survive of us is love.'

What secular Larkin cannot say is that our instinct is true, love survives. But what he must say, because of the power of this image and in fidelity to his first emotional response, is that it *feels* like that. This is a sensation that is felt by us all from time to time and one would have to be peculiarly foolish or insensitive to attempt to deny its reality. Of course, in one sense the reality is that of art, not of love itself but of its expression. This, however, does not diminish the effect of *feeling* the possibility. Indeed, the art could not exist without this possibility. It is not so much that we want the survival of love to be true, rather that there is something deep within us that remains stubbornly convinced that it is. Larkin's poem is art, as is the tomb, not because it offers wish-fulfilment but because it captures a truth that could not be expressed in any other way. As Unamuno saw, love and eternity are *necessarily* not contingently connected.

This is a commonplace of folk and popular culture. Loving couples give each other 'eternity' rings and lovers' vows are exchanged that could only ever be persuasive if they are deemed to be forever. 'A diamond is forever', runs the De Beers advertising line. And, in *Ghost* and *Titanic* (James Cameron 1997) and countless other movies, the message is pumped out that love is stronger than death.

Only love has this status among our emotions. In fact, precisely because it has this status, it is not seen as an emotion at all. Rather it is presented as a rock-like fact, something that crashes down upon us; it is not, like ordinary emotions, something that wells up from within. Or possibly it is a well, but one into which we dive – as in falling in love. Or it falls on us like a blessing, as in the love of children. In all cases, it is an event in the world, not just in ourselves, and it is this externality that is seen to validate its claim on eternity. This applies both to erotic and non-erotic love. Both gives us an irreducible interest in the persistence of the other through time.

Perversely perhaps, this becomes a problem when we are confronted with medical immortality. It is one thing to vow love to someone forever when that is unlikely to mean more than a few decades, quite another when it might mean hundreds of years. Could we possibly be serious in saying such a thing? Could we even believe such a thing about love for a child? Is it not possible that the eternity necessarily connected with love is the eternity of death? As Roger Scruton puts it, 'we love dying things'. Hence the difference between our conception of a flower that must die and one that cannot. The latter is no longer a flower at all, it has become something else, something we, as we are, would find hard if not impossible to love.

Let's Roll

'Are you guys ready? Let's roll.'

These were the last recorded words of Todd Beamer on 11 September 2001. What followed was a struggle with the terrorists who had hijacked United Airlines Flight 93 intending to crash it into Washington DC. The plane dived into the ground in Somerset County, Pennsylvania, harmlessly as far as the White House or the Capitol were concerned, but fatally for the terrorists, Beamer and the other passengers. In the United States, the words have become emblematic of heroism. Colloquial and masculine, they carry an acceptance of risk and a determination to act. The words have come to represent, to the American imagination, their country at its finest, rolling forward courageously into an uncertain future.

I mention them here because, though much of the science of the new immortality is being done outside of the US, all of the determination to roll the idea forward is American. Aubrey de Grey, the leading British figure in this world, happily acknowledges that Michael West, an American entrepreneur and scientist, is his mentor and role model. And, if West had a motto, it would be 'Let's Roll'.

To most of the Americans I have spoken to about this issue, any qualms about human life extension are mere quibbles. Conversations tend to follow the same pattern – 'Well, I guess that's true, but, come on, you'd take the pill, wouldn't you?' The quibbles are fine but if you take the pill you can go on having the argument; if you don't, you can't. Survival is the only game in town, it's the next big project, the next thing we must do after conquering the West, space and communism. It is an American event.

It was Benjamin Franklin, a great American technophile, who said, 'All that stands between us and eternal life are fear and gullibility. Dread of the unknown forges faith in the unknowable.' Franklin imagined it would be nice to be preserved – pickled – so as to be resurrected in the future, just as Alcor in Phoenix now freezes its patients in the hope that technology may one day be able to thaw and resurrect them. Cryonics is a very American idea, replete with a kind of literalness and an expression of the conviction that there must be a technical fix that will eliminate death. 'Deep down,' a New York friend once said to me, 'Americans think that death is optional.'

Above all, Americans regard death as an affront to their faith in the future. This faith is so strong that it seems to transform other, more conventional faiths. Two of the more startling discoveries I made in the course of working on this book were that Joe Waynick, chief executive of Alcor, is a Seventh Day Adventist, and David Gobel, founder of the Methuselah Foundation which supports research in longevity, is a Jehovah's Witness. Only Americans, I thought, could so smoothly combine such a secular goal as medical immortality with such fundamentalist belief systems.

The ancient Greeks called it *pleonexia*, the wish for more or, less attractively, greed. The Americans want more in a way that can never be completely satisfied and death is the supreme affront to that urge. It is, therefore, their pleonectic wish to get as much life and as little death as possible. The new immortality when/if it arrives will be an expression of the American dream.

Writing in 1965, the sociologist Robert Fulton glimpsed the peculiarly American nature of a new attitude towards death. 'In America today . . . we are beginning to react to death as we would to a communicable disease. Death is no longer viewed as the price of moral trespass or as the result of theological wrath; rather . . . death is coming to be seen as the consequence of personal neglect or untoward accident.'

Fulton was anticipating a transformation in the human imagination that matches the scientific transformation I have described in our view of the human body. It is a move from the idea of death as absolute and inevitable to the idea of death as something that must and can be avoided by the application of technology.

Four years later, in 1969, an American, Alan Harrington, one of the many counter-cultural heroes of that age, published a book called *The Immortalist: An Approach to the Engineering of Man's Divinity*. 'Death', announces Harrington on the first page, 'is an imposition on the human race, and no longer acceptable. Man has all but lost his ability to accommodate himself to personal extinction; he must now proceed physically to overcome it. In short, to kill death: to put an end to his own mortality . . .'

At one level, the book is very typical of its time. Like many others in the sixties Harrington was convinced that a new age had dawned in which old conflicts had no part. And it was precisely this banishing of old conflicts, that had exposed death itself as our true enemy. He writes: 'One of the advantages of having a cause is that it saves you from worrying about what life means . . . Only when the battle has ended does the freed soul turn and face the cosmic menace.'

But, at another level, the book is brilliantly prescient. Harrington sees, for example, that technology may be about to bring us to a turning point, a moment at which we can become gods. He also saw that this moment placed his generation in an awkward spot: 'We are caught between the desire to press home the final attack on the gods and the still-desperate need to placate them. We hang in doubt because we are the transitional people. The palace of immortality glitters in the distance. Who can be sure that our grandchildren will not live in it? But the near-certainty is that we will die, with the prospect of eternal life just out of reach.'

Harrington also had a solution for the problem of boredom – 'A state of indefinite living can be programmed through a succession of lives by means of designed sleeps or hibernations to last for years, decades or centuries.' And he anticipated Aubrey de Grey's 'escape velocity' argument – 'Today, if you can buy fifty years, you may look forward to more than a prayer of buying eternity.' Above all, he stated the primary immortalist creed that extending life indefinitely was no more than an extrapolation of conventional medicine: 'The truth is, of course, that death should no more be considered an acceptable part of life than smallpox or polio, both of which we have managed to bring under control without denouncing ourselves as presumptuous.'

Harrington was a true sixties radical, not a weekend hippie. His thought was couched in the most ambitious terms and was based on the conviction that this was not just an amelioration of the human condition he was proposing, it was a transformation. Immortality, like dodging the Vietnam draft, was both a right and an obligation. It was a case of hell no, we won't go gentle into that good night. It was the first statement of the baby-boomer discovery of death and, as the science writer Stephen S. Hall has observed, 'This is a generation, it goes without saying, that thinks of its petitions as somewhat special, a generation that is a little more insistent about answered prayers.'

This generation, of course, is the one that is now leading the medical assault on mortality. It is a generation of individualists, of course, and, as Josef Pieper has said, 'the more consciously man lives as an individual, the less he is capable of ignoring death'. And, as Feuerbach anticipated in the nineteenth century, we live in an age in which 'pure, naked personhood is considered to be the only substantial reality'.

It is, equally, a generation of technophiles and technocrats, a generation that believes things are fixable. Death must be fixable because, as Carol Zaleski puts it, death 'signals the failure of our medical technology, the evaporation of our dream of progress and self-fulfilment'.

But, in practice, Harrington's god-defying dreams were technologically premature and his message for the boomers was pessimistic. It was their grandchildren who would taste immortality rather than themselves. There were, however, some things they could do, some things they could buy. The debauch of the sixties – though it often did include macrobiotic (long life) foods – had been, in some ways, a death trip. The politically committed flung themselves at guns and clubs and the lotus eaters flung themselves at drugs.

In the seventies, some of the futile aspects were replaced by the healthier but less counter-cultural pose of expressing one's individuality through the pursuit of health. This may have been a step back from the transcendent ambitions of Harrington, but it was consistent with his view of survival as the only serious goal.

Here it is worth noting that the sixties – and, therefore, boomer – radicalism is closely associated with the pursuit of medical immortality. This radicalism is directed at the denial of full self-realisation of the people by authorities either wishing to maintain control of medicine or lacking in the imagination to give science a blank cheque to extend people's lives. The assumption is that the government will only recommend what it thinks people are capable of achieving. This may fall far short of optimum life-extension strategies and, therefore, self-actualisers that we are, it is up to us to seize the day.

Ray Kurzweil and Terry Grossman's book *Fantastic Voyage* is a reassertion of the sixties faith that we can transcend all our limitations. There is one important difference, however – these authors have absolute conviction that in the twenty-first century eternal life is visible on the horizon. 'The knowledge exists,' writes Kurzweil, 'if aggressively applied, for you to slow down aging and disease processes to such a degree that you can be in good health and good spirits when the more radical life extending and life enhancing technologies become available over the next couple of decades.'

Perhaps the tone of conviction is simply a matter of timing – Grossman and Kurzweil are boomers, both in their mid-fifties and, therefore, on the very edge of the possibility of dying just before the technology becomes available if the most optimistic projections are correct. *Fantastic Voyage* is bewildering in its range of recommendations. And the advice is given with a more pressing tone than anything that had gone before. Kurzweil and Grossman are advocating a huge effort but this time with the promise that, one day, the work will be over and earthly eternity is attainable. It must be a risk worth taking. It's the only game in town. Let's roll!

About Me (2)

The only time I feel, with any degree of rationality, immortal is when I am in Venice. There is nothing contrived about this feeling. I do not wish it upon myself. It is just there the moment I step ashore. It is not the immortality of not dying. I can well imagine my death in Venice, it almost happened once when I slipped and fell badly on the steps of the Rialto. It is, rather, the immortality of being part of a story told in the absolute worldly physicality of the stones, water and, of course, paint of this city. This may not be actual, personal survival, but it is real nonetheless, a unique sense of, as it were, outliving myself. I do not experience the same sensation in London, New York, Paris or in any city I have visited, only in Venice.

This is easily dismissed as self-dramatisation and perhaps it is. Or it may simply be said that great things have happened in my life in Venice – they have – therefore I feel unusually at home there. This is simply wrong, I don't feel remotely at home there; indeed, the immortal feeling has about it the, to me, pleasant quality of the alien and the solitary.

No, what I think I feel is the extraordinary unity of the place. Venice has many works of art, but Venice *is* one work of art. It is the only work of art in which one can live (and die) and the immortality it confers is that of art. Sometimes this seems to be enough.

4

Belonging, Heaven and Other Fixes

About Me (3)

My mother was Jewish. I did not discover this until I was about thirteen as she was very anti-Semitic. My father was an observant Anglican, though I am not sure of his true religious beliefs. He certainly believed in science and engineering. My wife is Catholic and I joined her church not long after we married. Many people think I am a Buddhist. This is because there is a prominent British Buddhist called Bryan Appleyard. He is not, however, me.

I acquired an anger with God from Judaism, a love of language from Anglicanism and a reverence for seriousness from Catholicism. From none did I acquire faith, though I was sure that there was something hidden behind the world of our senses, something that we could glimpse, but not necessarily know. An aspect of my Jewish anger with God was the way in which His world seemed to tantalise us with more than we could ever know. He promised us things He would never deliver – not least, immortality. Even in my most childishly earnest religious moments, in the depths of my private theology, I think I suspected my idea of immortality was not a faith but a fantasy. I still carry that fantasy within me, a faintly shameful survival of my childhood, which, like a weakness for sherbert dips, is not something to be discussed.

But, though without faith or hope, I did understand the religious impulse. It is the height of rationality to be struck dumb by the strangeness of my existence and of myself and the summit of irrationality to believe we can subdue such responses with mere reason. In that light, my own pessimistic lack of faith is a small matter. To me the simple polarity of belief-disbelief is a form of contemporary fundamentalism and explains why aggressively secular disbelievers find the world so hard to understand. I am religiously inclined and I accept religion. This makes me faithless and hopeless but religious.

I never conceived of immortality as a necessary aspect of religion. Almost from the beginning, I apprehended the immortality of the liturgy as essentially poetic. It moved me not as a serious promise or possibility, but, rather, as a statement that peace could be attained through these observances. And, especially in the Canticle of Simeon, the Nunc Dimittis of the English liturgy – 'Lord, now lettest thou thy servant depart in peace' – I did find peace. Peace is the one religious aspiration that has stayed with me always.

All of which puts me utterly out of step with conventional modern thought. Contemporary fundamentalism not only derives its faith from the glib trumping of belief by disbelief, it also delights in vulgar lampoons of the dreams of the faithful. These can be crude – why should you want to eat and drink the flesh and blood of your God? – or they can be slightly more subtle – don't you see that immortality is just a cheap bribe to make you accept oppression in this world, or that it is nothing but a consoling infantile fantasy? Having established this last – and, in their minds, crucial – point, the secular fundamentalists think they have finally destroyed religion. Having failed, as I said, to make the necessary connection between religion and immortality, this has always struck me as ridiculous.

The Bribe

Though I do have to accept that, strictly speaking, the word 'immortal' must be religious in that it denotes a being that cannot die. A medical immortal can easily die if he is hit by a truck, drowns or if the world is destroyed by some cosmic event. A true immortal would, by definition, survive all of these things and cannot, therefore, be a part of the material world. Even if we weaken immortality to the point where it simply means surviving in memory or mythology – like their heroes to the Greeks or Shakespeare and Mozart to us – the idea still cannot hold. The destruction of the earth would also entail the destruction of memory and, indeed, the physical destruction of literature and music. Any conception of true immortality must, therefore, involve the existence of an alternative, eternal world immune from the hazards of this one. A belief in such a world, for many, defines religion.

Our contemporary conception of immortality springs from this idea of religion as a way to survive death. It is a view held by believers and non-believers alike as the *sine qua non* of faith. To me, it has always been slightly shocking. I remember recoiling in horror when a Catholic priest said of a recently dead woman, 'I am sure she has gone straight to Heaven.' I felt that her post-mortem location was none of his business and well beyond his competence to determine. But, more importantly, I felt distaste for such literalness and, perhaps, some small pang of guilt that it exposed my own inability to believe. Yet I know that such literalness is exactly what many of the religious expect to hear and exactly what the secular find most absurd about their faith.

In fact, the full secular orthodoxy goes much further than this. Survival of death is not just an absurd idea in itself, it is also the complete explanation of religion, its origins and its persistence. People, they argue, are so afraid of death that they invent consoling afterlife fantasies and systematise these fantasies into religions. The motives of Islamic suicide bombers are felt to be fully explained by the fact that they go to their death convinced they are taking a short cut to paradise. Basically, this is a way of seeing religion solely as a crude bribe, an offer of post-mortem rewards to compensate for sufferings in this life or for the fact of death.

This idea has distinguished champions who turned it into a secular orthodoxy. Karl Marx saw religion as part of the apparatus of oppression, 'the opium of the masses', which persuaded people to endure suffering in this life in the hope of an eternity of happiness and comfort in the next. Sigmund Freud saw religion as an infantile disorder, a dysfunctional inability to face reality. People, he argued, do not truly believe in their own mortality and so they create compensatory myths. Sir James Frazer, the influential social anthropologist, concluded that 'the gist of the whole story of the fall appears to be an attempt to explain man's mortality, to set forth how death came into the world'. From politics, psychology and comparative religion came the same conclusion – immortality was a bribe, the central comforting delusion provided by religion. The Polish anthropologist Bronislaw Malinowski summarised this sense that religion had somehow been explained away. He wrote: 'Survival after death is probably one of the earliest mythical hypotheses, related perhaps to some deep biological craving of the organism, but certainly contributing to the stability of social groups and towards the sense that human endeavours are not as limited as purely rational experience shows.'

Doubtless, immortality is, indeed, a comforting delusion for many religious people; doubtless, these theories have some explanatory power in reinforcing that view. But there are two big problems with the bribe theory: first, it may explain why some people are religious but not why so many are and have been and, secondly, it is entirely unsupported by evidence.

These thinkers did not have evidence, they simply argued that it must be so, therefore it is so. In fact, what evidence there is points the other way. The origins of religion may well lie in attempts to give meaning to death, but they certainly do not lie in attempts to provide immortal rewards. Neither the early Jews, who believed in a shadowy existence in Sheol after death, nor the Ancient Greeks, who believed in a similarly tenuous stay in Hades, regarded the afterlife as any kind of reward. Hinduism and Buddhism speak of reincarnation, but seldom of the literal self, more exactly as the continuance of karma, the chain of cause and effect of which the individual was but one small part. Equally, we do not know what the flowers left in the graves of the middle Palaeolithic era signified. People casually take them to mean some sort of continuity, but disbelievers put flowers on graves today as a sign of memory, not as a sign of the survival of the dead. And it is not necessarily the case that the placing of the goods of a dead man alongside him in his grave was done to aid him in the afterlife. They could equally well have been a way of removing him more completely from the realm of the living. Historically, it has been a common impulse to regard the dead as a threat and to remove them from contact with the society of the living. And, finally, humans do not need the promise of immortality as a reason to blow themselves up. In

Sri Lanka the Tamil Tigers, anti-religious Leninists, until recently were responsible for more suicide bombings than any other group. Religion may be about the continuance of things, but it is not necessarily about the literal continuance of the self. And, if it is not, then the bribe theory collapses.

This contemporary delusion that religion is and always has been concerned with personal survival after death hinges on the word 'personal'. The arguments of Marx, Freud and Frazer only work if we see religion as offering the actual survival of the self. The bribe on offer is that I will survive death intact, that I shall find myself on the other side to be much the same as I am on this side – either as a spirit or as an embodied being. Such an offer is, in fact, very rare in the history of religion. Buddhism, seeing the self as an illusion, makes no such offer and neither does Hinduism. Indeed, in both cases, the supreme religious goal is seen as release from the prison of the self. Judaism sometimes does and sometimes doesn't. At the time of Christ, the Sadducees denied an afterlife while the Pharisees believed in an afterlife of punishments and rewards. But, for all Jews, the primary form of immortality on offer is not personal but as a part of the story of Israel. Nationally based faiths like Shinto offer the same kind of consolation. Pericles offered the Athenians of the Golden Age something similar in his great funeral oration for the war dead – 'For in magnifying the city I have magnified them, and men like them whose virtues made her glorious.' Personal survival is either not on offer at all or only to a limited few through much of Christian history. The religions of ancient Greece and Rome may have offered Hades a continued existence as a feeble shadow, or something slightly more consoling, but seldom with any consistency. Islam, the most recent and the most literal of the monotheistic faiths, alone seems to have been consistent in promising personal survival.

The modern idea that personal immortality is all that religions have ever offered is, therefore, plainly mistaken. The
mistake happens because of a desire to project back into the
past the contemporary conception of the self as the ultimate reality, the only possible object of value, and
self-actualisation as the only worthwhile project. Religions
do consistently say that something continues, but it is
seldom the self as it is currently understood. So, in reality,
the history of religion should not be seen as the pursuit of
personal immortality, but rather as the search for belonging,
meaning and value.

'It is', writes the theologian John Bowker, 'an exploration
of how value can be maintained at the limit of life without
seeking illusory compensation.'

In this context, there is an ambivalence about the contemporary pursuit of medical immortality. It can be seen as an
extension of the faith of scientism. The belief in the omni-
competence of science necessarily involves the conviction that
it can make the human body – and that is understood to
include the self – medically immortal. Or it can be seen as
the logical continuation of the contemporary pursuit of self-
actualisation, a project which is inevitably hampered by the
relative brevity of the existence of the self. The overcoming of
this problem of brevity can be seen, as it is by many immortalists, as consistent with the Western Enlightenment tradition
of placing ultimate value on the individual life.

Or it can be seen, rather startlingly, by some very religious
people as entirely consistent with the wishes of the Christian
God. Alcor's former chief executive Joe Waynick, for example, came to the conclusion, in conversations with his pastor,
that cryonics was an entirely legitimate pursuit: 'We both
came to the conclusion that there is no biblical reason why
you cannot participate in a cryonics experiment any more
than one could not participate in a heart transplantation or

take experimental drugs. It's a medical treatment like any other.'

Dave Gobel, founder of the Methuselah Foundation which promotes life-extension technologies, found a similar way to reconcile his faith with technology: 'I don't believe there is an afterlife for most people. Genesis says from dust you are and to dust you will return . . . When we die we go back to the Earth. I also believe God can reconstitute human beings or things if he chooses to. We can reboot computers. To me coming back to life would be like rebooting.'

Contemporary immortalism is plainly a broad church. On the other hand, these disparate views can be united under two banners – we place ultimate value on individual lives and life extension is a medical treatment like any other. Beneath these banners, neither humanist nor religious values are mocked by the search for technologies of life extension. Yet neither are they asserted, for merely extending the duration of the self does not give it meaning or value. The awkward truth is that only religion can do that.

Belonging

Madame de Montespan, mistress of Louis XIV, had a horror of dying alone. When in bed, she kept the curtains open and insisted on being surrounded by lit candles and women chatting. If the women fell asleep, she would wake them. When she finally realised her death really was approaching on 27 May 1707, she summoned all her servants and, in the words of Philippe Aries, 'presided, as was the custom, over the ceremony of her own death'.

There is something terrible about dying alone, even when you want to die. A recent news story tells me that the Japanese have taken to group suicides. Police report that ninety-one 'strangers afraid to die alone' had died in the company of others in 2005. They used the Internet to find others with the same desire. Group suicides do seem to persuade people of the wisdom or necessity of the act. At Jonestown, Guayana, in 1978, 913 members of the People's Temple, a Christian cult formed around James Warren Jones, drank cyanide on his instructions. And in 1997, 39 members of the Heaven's Gate cult were found dead in San Diego. There are many such examples; a group seems to make death more palatable.

What is wrong with dying alone? On the face of it, one has no choice in the matter. Even if you are surrounded by other dying people, the act itself is necessarily a solitary, introspective business. Being surrounded by chatting women would seem to be no help. But, in fact, I think it would. I hate all medical procedures, particularly those involving my own unconsciousness. On one occasion I was given a general anaesthetic for a minor operation and, as I was about to slip under, I felt a wave of panic. A nurse, perhaps spotting this, stroked my brow; at once the panic vanished and I succumbed happily. Doubtless, it is a gesture devoid of any special feeling, a procedure advocated by wise and experienced teachers. But it worked. I have, ever since, felt strongly that it would also have worked if I had been dying.

The stroked brow and the chatting women provide the consolation not simply that we are not alone but that we belong to a human community. Both evoke what we have in common, as social creatures and as anxious, vulnerable beings. Furthermore, when Madame de Montespan actually did die, she did so in public in the manner of her time. Deathbeds in those days were customarily attended by family and friends. They did not, as we tend to do, conceal this last rite of passage in a hospital ward. These are the consolations of belonging, of being a part of a continuity. To truly belong is to be reconciled to life and, thereby, to death.

The core appeal of religion is its offer of belonging. Whatever else might define our membership of a given community – language, race, land – religion remains the most potent sign that we are not alone. Hinduism joins the faithful to the great wheel of existence, Christianity to the body of Christ, Islam to the Umma, the worldwide body of believers, and Buddhism to the common pursuit of the enlightenment offered by the wisdom of the Buddha. Roman Catholics often speak of baptism, the first of the seven sacraments, as putting a mark on the soul, a badge of membership visible only to God. Of course, for some religious people – the contemplative, the saint at odds with his world and his time – not belonging is the badge and the pursuit of solitary ecstasy is the clearest mark of faith. But, for most, the meaning religion offers is communal both in space – here in this church or temple – and time – at one with those who have gone before and will come after. Through belonging, as Zygmunt Bauman put it, we privatise death and collectivise immortality.

This sense of belonging is, far more than any concept of personal immortality, the primordial aspect of religion. This is because of the depth of loneliness that is intrinsic to the human condition. It is the fact of loneliness, not death, that is most shocking about our time on earth. By loneliness I mean here the feeling of being disconnected, of having no home.

'Why is the human a spiritual being?' asked Ludwig Feuerbach. 'Not just because he is distinct from nature, but because his distinction from nature is a result of his own activity of distinguishing. The human by nature is distinguished from nature . . .'

We may know that, like the animals we are, we belong to nature. But the problem is the knowing. We are the attainment of self-consciousness by nature, but that very attainment cuts us off from the comfort of being entirely in nature. We cannot help but distinguish ourselves from unself-conscious life and, as Feuerbach sees, that act evicts us from our natural home. And so we construct various spiritualities – systems bigger than ourselves – to replace the system we have lost. When religion offers belonging, it offers a solution to the problem of self-awareness.

The form of this solution varies wildly but, at its most basic, belonging simply means what it says. The belonging to the state, race or creed is all that people need to transcend the crisis of their loneliness. Thus both ancient Jewish and Greek religion began with a very unattractive view of an afterlife as enfeebled ghosts – in Hades for the Greeks and Sheol for the Jews – and then converged on the idea that all that really mattered was the individual's place in the story of Athens or Israel. This is, of course, not *all* that was involved in these religions, but it is a crucial and, for much of the time, dominant strand in both.

Immortality is achieved not by the individual but by the community. The same sort of self-sublimation appears to have occurred in Inca religion and it is intrinsic to Shinto. Although the latter is an animistic belief that sees the world as suffused with billions of spirits – *kami* – and, indeed, on death we join those spirits, it is a system that depends on the story of Japan as the uniquely blessed abode of both humans and spirits. Shinto requires not belief but ritual as a way of fitting us to life in this world.

The Romans took their own primary concept of immortality from the Greeks. The foundation of the city was the supremely sacred moment and all succeeding generations were saved by continuing the story of that foundation. The authority of Rome was derived from tradition and thus from memory. It is no accident, as Hannah Arendt pointed out, that the two most distinctively Roman divinities were Janus – the god of beginnings who still survives in our language as

January – and Minerva – the goddess of wisdom and memory, two effectively interchangeable virtues. The duty of keeping the past alive in memory is, both to the Romans and to us, a religious injunction.

This kind of immortality may seem a little thin to the contemporary imagination. Yet it remains a potent force for the obvious reason that it provides very clear, simple, undemanding consolation to the living and to the dying by linking individual death to communal continuance. As a result, this immortality of communal belonging echoes down the ages. The funeral oration of Pericles, which defined the immortality of the citizens of Athens, is precisely echoed in Abraham Lincoln's Gettysburg Address, a speech he delivered in 1863 during the American Civil War. Lincoln, in fact, goes further than Pericles in insisting on the power of the dead over the living and, therefore, over the future. He speaks of the people gathered there to dedicate a cemetery and then adds:

> But, in a larger sense, we can not dedicate – we can not consecrate – we can not hallow – this ground. The brave men, living and dead, who struggled here, have consecrated it, far above our poor power to add or detract. The world will little note, nor long remember what we say here, but it can never forget what they did here. It is for us the living, rather, to be dedicated here to the unfinished work which they who fought here have thus far so nobly advanced.

The living cannot add to what the dead have done, nor can they take anything away. The acts of the dead cannot be undone. The dead have become a necessary part of any future story and, therefore, immortal. Most familiarly, to the British at least, this idea appears in the fourth stanza of Laurence Binyon's 1914 poem 'For the Fallen':

They shall grow not old, as we that are left grow old:
Age shall not weary them, nor the years contemn.
At the going down of the sun and in the morning
We will remember them.

Note that Binyon adds to the Pericles–Lincoln theme the contemporary idea that dying young saves the heroes from the
miseries of old age. This step brings the idea of heroic com-
munality into our own time. Remove the military heroism
and replace it with contemporary self-actualisation and you
have the rock 'n' roll ideal of living fast, dying young and
leaving a beautiful corpse. This is partly a hip joke, of course,
but only partly. Pop cultural heroes like James Dean, Jim
Morrison, Jimi Hendrix, Janis Joplin and Kurt Cobain represent a particular form of heroism and possess a degree of
immortality in memory precisely because they died young. At
the climax of Oliver Stone's film *The Doors* (1991), this
transfiguring power of the good rock death is made explicit.
The corpse of Jim Morrison is shown to have regained the
youth and beauty which the living body had lost through the
usual mix of drugs and debauchery. The premature death
redeems the rock star as it did the boy in the trenches, keeping them both forever young.

   Yet this idea of the heroic immortals cannot necessarily
redeem the community of which they are a part. There are,
after all, evil communities. As Zygmunt Bauman has
pointed out, 'Construction of group immortality can be
interpreted as an attempt to harness the energy generated by
death-anxiety in the service of specific group interests and,
of course, the interests of the group's extant or aspiring
elites.'

   In other words, it may be all very well to die for Athens,
Rome, the Union, Britain or even rock 'n' roll, but it is not
quite the same to die for Stalin, Hitler or Tojo. Evil dictators

and unjust wars would seem to consign their heroic dead not to immortality but oblivion.

But, then again, why? The Nuremberg Trials (1945–1949) of Nazi war criminals established the idea of individual guilt within the context of a collective action. In the West, we have come to accept the idea that some kinds of death may be accorded the blessed immortality of national memory, but others may not. Yet this can be seen as irrational or even unjust. After all, the individual soldier on any side, fighting for any country, is unlikely to know as he goes into battle whether history will see the cause for which he offers his life as good or bad. Or – a stronger version of the same point – true virtues lies in the act of dying for the nation, not in any moral evaluation of the country's posture at the time.

The Japanese have – though they seldom say so explicitly – refused to accept the Western consensus on war guilt. For them, either the weak version of the argument is sustained by the conviction that their role in the Second World War was to drive Western imperialists from Asia, or the strong version is sustained by the belief in the special destiny of Japan. All of this is focused on the Yasukuni (Peaceful Nation) Shrine in Tokyo. Some 2.5 million *kami* of the country's war dead are said to reside here. Unfortunately, fourteen of them are regarded as high grade war criminals by the West. That fact alone discredits the shrine for Westerners, though not for most Japanese. Of course, the *kami* of the heroic dead are still literally alive in this world. But this aspect is not the primary point about Yasukuni. The heart of the matter is the duty of the living to honour the fallen as immortals because of their part in the story of Japan. From Pericles to Yasukuni, the conferring of immortality through the mechanism of the communal narrative has maintained its grip on the human imagination. At Yasukuni it is as potent as ever.

Over the last 200 years in the West, it has been elaborated

further by the conception of history itself as a redeeming narrative. In this version, the nation is suppressed in favour of a
global destiny. From Hegel through Marx and down to various contemporary utopianisms of both the left and right, the
modern mind has attempted to escape from the chaos of the
present and the crisis of individual death into the quasi-time-
less generality of an unfolding narrative of history. Typically,
we are seen as treading an upward path leading to a brighter
future. We are redeemed simply by the fact that we keep to
this path. In most liberal interpretations, this future is merely
seen as somewhat better than the present. But tougher ide-
ologies see it as absolutely better, believing there is a final
state of humanity in which all our problems will be solved.
Either way, the upward path redeems the life since, as Arendt
puts it, 'no matter how haphazard single actions may appear
in the present and in their singularity, they inevitably lead to
a sequence of events forming a story that can be rendered
through intelligible narrative the moment the events are
removed into the past'.

This is not a remote, intellectual concept, it is a way of life.
Years ago I recognised its power when, after a drunken night,
some hard Marxist student friends parted company with my
own ideologically vaguer group.

'Where are you going?' I called across the street.

One of the Marxists thrust his fist into the air. 'Where the
struggle leads us!'

He was not joking. It was, for me, an epiphany, a revelation of an utterly different type of imagination, one that saw
a continuous flow of meaning and justification in every event
and in every individual action. This would, of course, also
have been true of a good Christian imagination – that faith
also defines a view of history ending in some perfected state
and endows every moment of life with transcendent significance – but the lukewarm Christianity of post-war Britain

had shown my student self no examples of lives lived in the light of such certainty. I could not imagine any of the clergy I had known yelling in the street with such conviction. In my Marxist friend's cry, I had glimpsed the reality of ordinary time redeemed by faith. I was impressed and scared.

I had good reason to be scared. In its harshest, Leninist form, Marxism was used as an excuse to devalue present life utterly. Both Stalin and Mao Tse-Tung, like Lenin before them, saw the deaths of millions as small matters in the light of the great projects on which they were engaged. In some routine rituals or memorials, these millions may have been acknowledged as workers in the great task, but the reality was that their deaths were seen as trivial, not necessary and sacrificial. They were simply an inevitable by-product of the process. One death, Stalin famously said, is a tragedy, a million are a statistic. A few people's present may be redeemed by the path to future perfection, but most people's lives were indistinguishable from industrial effluent.

The weaker, liberal form of the belief merely in a better future rather than in a perfect end state is, broadly speaking, the only faith of humanist secularity. As Albert Camus said, 'The future is the only transcendent value for men without God.' And so we have Bill Clinton telling us not to stop thinking about tomorrow and Tony Blair's New Labour saying 'forward not back'. The future is an unwritten book and it can, therefore, be better written than the present. It is pure, a blank page, and this purity is highly seductive to the contemporary imagination. Once, hurrying to catch a connecting flight in Newark airport in America, I was stopped in my tracks by a builder's sign that read: 'Forgive the inconvenience, we are knocking down yesterday to build tomorrow.' What startled me was the blithe assumption that everybody would agree that this was a virtuous project. But, of course, they do because of the secular, humanist faith in the future.

It is a faith based, in essence, on the discovery of a form of human knowledge – science – that is cumulative and on the experience of two centuries of continuous economic growth in the countries that have applied the wisdom of science most effectively through technological innovation. The central doctrine of this faith is twofold: first the accumulation of knowledge and that its application will continue and, secondly, this continuing accumulation will lead to a continuing improvement in the human condition. And so if we have a problem now – cancer, global warming – it will be fixed in the future.

Plainly there is much that is arguable about this faith and, equally plainly, it *is* a faith as there can be no evidence that accumulation and improvement can continue. But, leaving such doubts aside, this is the faith from which now springs the pursuit of medical immortality. So the religion of belonging, which became, in the modern era, the religion of belonging to history, finally moves from the immortality not of the individual self but of the self's place in history to an aspiration for actual immortality of the self. Enfolded in the doctrine of progress, the immortalists seek to crown their faith with the ultimate reward.

In our period – roughly the last hundred years – the progressive faith combined with the growing force of the belief in the cultivation of the self has produced a further variation on the theme of immortality through belonging. This began as the star system and became the celebrity system. Effectively, this was born in 1910 in Hollywood when Carl Laemmle poached an actress then only known as the Biograph Girl from Biograph Studios. Silent movie stars had, until then, been anonymous. But the public curiosity about these people – as well as the deal this actress made with Laemmle – led to her rather odd name, Florence Lawrence, being made public. The star system was born.

Stars are different from celebrities. As James F. English has written, the celebrity system as opposed to the star system is based on 'a logic of exaggerated intimacy rather than exaggerated distance'. Stars were adored from afar and their lives were filtered through a thick gauze of studio control. Laemmle was able to enhance the impact of the naming of the Biograph Girl by spreading the rumour that she had been killed by an accident in New York, a device that would now be almost impossible thanks to the power and intrusiveness of the media. The lives of celebrities, in contrast, are lived on screen and in print. Public relations may still successfully manipulate what we know but, as English sees, the stories always offer intimacy, the feeling of the real presence of the person.

But offering a person in this way at all – whether intimately or at a distance – is made possible entirely by technology. It is one thing to hear tales of heroes or see them depicted in paintings or sculptures, quite another thing to see them walking and talking in front of your eyes even when they are not, in fact, there. Both the development of still photographs and moving pictures had momentous effects on the human imagination. The first convinced many that all other forms of representation had been rendered obsolete and the second disoriented people's sense of the real. One of the earliest films of the Lumière Brothers was *L'Arrivee d'un Train en Gare de La Ciotat*. It simply shows a train pulling into a station. When it was first shown in Paris, there was panic in the theatre. Pictures, in their minds, did not move; if they did move they must be real.

Few of us have fully lost this seemingly primitive sense that there is something uncanny about moving pictures. A century of cinema may have had the effect of embedding it more deeply in our imaginations. The actor who dies in one film only to be resurrected in another sustains the child's view that death must be simply one more event in life. But there is also plenty of recent evidence that adults continue to be confused. 'Reality' television is so-called because it seems to show real people in real situations. But, of course, both the situations and the people are rendered unreal by the presence of the cameras. The lens changes everything, leaves nothing quite where it was. As I write this a series of *Celebrity Big Brother* – a reality show that involves imprisoning a group of people, in this case, celebrities, in a house for three weeks – has just ended. The game is played by audience votes removing cast members they do not like. The joke of this series is that it was won by the one person who wasn't actually a celebrity. She was simply a pretty girl who was said to be a member of a pop group, though she wasn't. The democratic-seeming triumph was that she was shown to be more popular than the celebrity elite. Except that she was made a minor celebrity by being on the show and a slightly less minor one by winning it.

Stars and celebrities are the contemporary correlatives of the heroes and gods of the past. Like them, they are seen to inhabit a different realm from the rest of us. Even intimately perceived celebrities, as opposed to distantly perceived stars, inhabit a land that is more brilliant, more vivid than our own. Their closely observed human failings may say they are just like the rest of us, but precisely because they are so closely observed they are transformed by the lens into special, emblematic examples of our own failings. These people are sanctified by fame and the rest of us are sanctified by being the fame-givers; it is we who say they are famous. You cannot, after all, be famous alone. Fame is our Athens or Jerusalem, it is what gives us belonging. It makes the famous immortal and gives the rest of us a sense of belonging, allowing us, therefore, to partake of immortality.

There is, finally, one other, much more persuasive contemporary expression of the religion of belonging. In its current form it is expressed through environmentalism, though it is a very ancient idea. It can be found among the American Indians and the Australian Aborigines. In the form most familiar to me and in which it has been most vividly expressed both through science and art, it is English. It is probably true to say that the English – not the British – developed their idea of 'home', the place where they belong, from the Romans. As I have said, the Roman idea of belonging, of immortality, was derived from their sense of the story of their city, its foundation and subsequent greatness. Where they belonged, therefore, was geographically defined, not racially or any of the other ways in which people have explained their sense of home. The English maintained this geographical sense of belonging, perhaps because they too acquired a global empire, a foreign place which they could make look like home. The love of the specifically English landscape – the oak trees, the hills, the churches, the villages – remains a commonplace of our culture.

In its most exalted form, this love becomes an absolute form of belonging, a sense of unity with the land. This can be demonstrated by countless examples. Here is one. Humphrey Repton was a great English landscape gardener. He was born in 1752 and died in 1818. He is buried by the porch of Aylsham Church in Norfolk. This is the inscription over the grave:

> Not like Egyptian tyrants consecrate;
> Unmixed with others shall my dust remain;
> But mold'ring blending, melting into Earth;
> Mine shall give form and colour to the Rose;
> And while its vivid blossoms cheer Mankind,
> Its perfumed odours shall ascend to Heaven.

Repton wants his body to become one with the soil and

specifically opposes this wish to the desire of the pharaohs to
be, in death, set apart from all else. The pharaoh does not
belong, but Repton will because his body will sink into the
soil and be taken up by the rose to delight others and send
perfume to heaven.

This conception of immortality prefigures both the scientific shocks of the nineteenth century and the environmental
response to those shocks. The geology of James Hutton and
Charles Lyell revealed the world to be much older than religious accounts suggested it should be and the biology of
Charles Darwin revealed that there was nothing special about
human beings, we were born of the same system as all other
organisms. Such insights gradually eroded the literal foundations of faith and produced the very English pessimism of
writers like Matthew Arnold and Thomas Hardy.

But if nineteenth-century geology and biology separate us
from what we thought we were, they also endow us with a
new identity, make us characters in a new story. This might
be seen as the story of nature – it often is – but that is not
quite right. Nature, viewed as the entire cosmos, appears, to
a rough approximation, to be entirely dead. It is, rather, the
story of the earth and the thin film of life which it sustains.
Repton celebrates his sinking back into this commonality of
life after death. He does refer to heaven, but he does not
seem to take this to mean the survival of himself. Rather, he
rejects the harsh individuality of the pharaoh in favour of
what seems to be a loss of self, perhaps a blessed relief from
its sufferings.

This English conception of immortality has much in
common with eastern conceptions of life as reality and the
individual as a passing illusion. In our day, it has acquired a
scientific validation. James Lovelock, a very great independent English scientist and the deepest of deep greens, devised
the Gaia hypothesis. Named after the Greek goddess of the

earth, this viewed the earth as a single organism. This was based on his analysis of the way planetary systems – the salinity of the oceans, temperatures and so on – are regulated by life. Since all these systems were interconnected, they behaved as one gigantic unitary system. Originally, Lovelock insisted that Gaia was a metaphor but lately he seems to be saying that it is not, that the earth is a single organism.

But, metaphor or not, Lovelock's Gaia is indeed a goddess in that she reigns over us. Without her, we are nothing. Without us, she can continue to live a perfectly healthy existence. She did so in the billions of years in which the earth was alive before humans arrived. Gaia is, therefore, an external limit and discipline for our species. She defies both humanist conceptions of progress and our ability to create meaningful values and Christian conceptions of mankind's stewardship of nature.

Most importantly, she offers a scientifically detailed version of an immortality of belonging. We are as immortal as life on earth, no more and no less. If we destroy life on earth, as we might, then we destroy our own immortality. If we sustain Gaia, we sustain ourselves. We belong to life, the only life we know.

Heaven

Those who believe in religion as a bribe are usually referring to the idea of heaven, a place of bliss where we survive not as life in general but as ourselves or as improved versions of ourselves. Heaven is a reward which, to the unbeliever, is proffered the better to make us endure the hardships and privations of this life or to more willingly succumb to authority. But to the believer heaven is also a reward in that it is attained as the prize of a virtuous life.

The reward of heaven is bliss, of course, but more

fundamentally it is immortality. The whole point of heaven, for most people, is that it signals freedom from death. Since many if not all of the evils of this world are connected to ageing and death, then a heaven may simply be defined as a place where there is no death, irrespective of its other qualities. Of course, that much may be said of hell. But there the sufferings of this life are magnified and extended through eternity. Immortality for the damned is one further torture.

Heaven raises some fairly obvious questions. Where is it? What is it like? What do people do there? Are they people or just extracts of people, spirits that once inhabited bodies? And when do the virtuous get there – at the moment of death or much later, at the Day of Judgement?

The literalness of these questions may seem odd if, like me, you regard heaven as a poetic rather than an actual place or if you are simply a rank unbeliever. But that is to miss the sense in which human self-awareness seems not simply to expect or believe in heaven, but to *demand* it.

Even the most glowing optimist must acknowledge that life in this world is patchy. For every up there is a down and for every birth there is a death. 'Life is hard,' as the saying goes, 'then you die.' A difficulty is terminated by an outrage. And yet all the time there are these ups, these shafts of happiness which seem to be glimpses of perfection. Love, most commonly, suggests that this patchy existence can, indeed, be perfected if only we could always be in the first ecstasies of love. Surely such experiences are portents of a life we cannot yet have, a life elsewhere, a life beyond the grave.

But the body visibly rots after death. Conceivably it might be restored at some later date and that is, indeed, believed by many. Or it might be claimed that the rotting is some kind of illusion and the true body has, in fact, been transported elsewhere. But the most common device for describing what survives to experience heaven is the soul.

Exactly who first split the human being into body and soul is unclear but the idea was certainly present in Plato and it is Platonic thinking that suffuses the Western conception of the soul. It may be that every human has experienced some such intuition. As I said in describing my own experiences of death, the feeling that something has actually left the corpse is utterly persuasive. We would now say that what has departed is not a separable thing but rather something like the functional integrity of the whole system, the body has died as a car breaks down. But, prior to such machine metaphors, the fact of death would have convinced anybody that this flesh was actually inhabited by something which had now departed. In fact, one does not have to observe a corpse, one can sense the same thing through introspection. As our bodies change through our lives so do our minds but, apparently, not completely. Something inside me seems to be the same as it was ten, twenty or thirty years ago and will still be the same in the future. That something seems to be inhabiting the flesh rather than being at one with it.

There have been numerous other attempts to define the physical reality of the soul, perhaps the most familiar was spiritualism with which I shall deal in the next chapter. But, in practice, the existence of the soul did not, for most people, require such physical evidence. It was simply true, both introspectively and through faith. This self-evident quality makes the soul one of the few religious concepts that seems to survive intact in secular society. Most commonly, it is taken to mean emotional depth as in 'soul' music or any set of attributes that goes beyond purely material or practical considerations. If the word 'soul' were banned tomorrow, there would be an enormous hole left in the language. It is our way of expressing the feeling that consciousness, somehow, goes beyond the immediate world of our senses.

Heaven is an extension of this feeling. If we do have a soul that is separable from our bodies, then plainly it is not at ease in this world. Heaven would be a place where it was fully at ease, finally satisfied and at peace. This is easy to say, less easy to imagine. But we persist in the attempt. Human history could be rewritten as a history of heaven.

The 'bribe' idea of heaven as a reward for virtuous suffering in this world and the corresponding idea of hell as a punishment seems to have been embedded forever in the Western tradition by Plato, though he did not believe it himself. It was intended as a 'noble lie', a political tool to keep the masses in check. In this sense, the bribe theorists would seem to be right. And it is certainly true that the reward–punishment system in the afterlife would continue, long after Plato, to be used for political coercion. But, in fact, this shows the bribe theorists to be wrong because their theory was of religious origins. Plainly, if Plato consciously invented this idea, then it does not explain religion, only a use of it.

Whatever its role on earth, the central problem of heaven is obvious – the changeability of human desire and the brevity of human happiness. At different times, we have different ideas of what is most desirable. To the hungry man, food is heaven, to the thirsty, drink, to the lover, sex, and so on. And we are all hungry, thirsty or aroused from time to time. Even when we are fully satisfied in all aspects, we know that new distractions and desires will soon make us restless. Heaven would thus need to be a constantly changing form of bliss or some sort of total satisfaction we cannot imagine while trapped in these bodies.

The primary debate – in the Christian world at least – has been between those who favour a heaven full of people or one simply full of God, an anthropocentric or a theocentric paradise. The anthropocentric heaven may be seen as the most distinctive Christian innovation. Other versions of the afterlife tend to portray rather grim places like Sheol and Hades,

specialised warrior paradises or ineffable conditions of fulfil-
ment like Nirvana which may or may not be different from
oblivion. Or, of course, there is the extremely exclusive afterlife reserved for the pharaoh alone. But the novelty of the
Christian paradise is that it is open to all, as is the Christian
hell. Our souls are all equal before God and the final destinations of those souls are determined not by rank but by
character. Since it is character that is at stake, the heaven
that is implied is one in which our selves continue, liberated
by death from the trials and restrictions of this life. This produces the familiar medieval and Renaissance images of the
teeming multitudes in paradise and all subsequent images of
gardens, fountains, countryside and towns that show heaven
as an idealised version of the world we already know.

Yet heaven as more of the same in the garden of God still
raises difficult questions. We are already alive among our
loved ones and we remain ourselves here and now and yet we
do not seem to be satisfied. What is so different about our
state of mind in heaven that makes eternity seem bearable?
The answer was a complete rejection of this idea of heaven
and its replacement with a strongly theocentric vision. This
vision is necessarily more theoretical, more intellectual, as it
involves a consolation which we cannot imagine and which is
not based on the ordinary consolations of the here and now.
It is the vision of St Paul when he speaks of seeing 'through a
glass, darkly' and of the prospect of knowing 'even as also I
am known', a reference to the way the existence of the soul
turns our conscious, embodied selves into a code. But, most
persuasively, it is the vision of St Thomas Aquinas who created the idea of heaven not as a teeming paradise of reunions
and social activities, but as an eternity filled only with direct
knowledge of God.

This medieval heaven was, in fact, Aristotle's. Aquinas's
central contribution both to the Church and to Western

civilisation was the unification of classical and Christian wisdom. Aristotle provided the physics and cosmology that, after Aquinas, who died in 1274, was to be the Christian orthodoxy until its undermining by Galileo in the early seventeenth century. At the heart of this orthodoxy was a highly specific conception of stillness. Our world is full of change and movement. The observable universe, however, is not. As we move away from our planet, matter becomes ever more still, changeless and perfect. We now know, of course, that the universe is full of constant and violent change. But to know this requires detailed and lengthy observation as well as telescopes. Before Galileo, the fixed and unchangeable heavens were not so much a faith as an accepted fact.

Perfection, therefore, was unchangeable and, because movement must involve change, immobile. To turn this into a satisfactory idea of heaven, the Aristotelian concept of happiness is also required. This is an entirely intellectual condition, far beyond any satisfactions of the senses. Contemplation is the ideal. Thus, for Aquinas, heaven is the still, unchanging contemplation of God.

This was difficult to imagine and so, predictably, the modern era saw the rebirth of the anthropocentric idea of heaven, specifically in the writings of the Swedish mystic Swedenborg in the eighteenth century. Once again, heaven was seen as a place of human reunion and human delights. This was the consoling story told throughout the nineteenth and into the early twentieth century, at which point it began to be superseded by a new form of the scholarly, contemplative heaven defined by the leading Protestant theologians.

With the French Revolution and the Romantic movement, an anthropocentric modernity was born. It was far from being godless – the revolutionaries instituted a Festival of the Supreme Being – but it rejected orthodox hierarchies and most of the conventional, institutionalised trappings of

Christianity. Rather, it reverted to a Platonism of an idealised other world, from which, in the terms of the supreme romantic William Wordsworth, we arrived on earth 'trailing clouds of glory' and to which, after our trials in this life, we would return.

The conflict between the theocentric and the anthropocentric heaven continues today. The theocentric view persists in various forms of mysticism and in the high, intellectual theology of thinkers like Karl Barth and Karl Rahner. On the other hand, there is the extreme literalism of radical Islam with its belief in instant sensory rewards for the suicide bombers who die righteous deaths. Or there is contemporary American fundamentalism based on the literal truth of the Book of Revelations. In this, modern geopolitical events – notably the foundation of the state of Israel and the imminent appearance of the anti-Christ in the form of a European leader – are seen as the preparatory signs of the end time.

Both Islamic and Christian fundamentalists insist on the actual physical reality of what will occur after death. They do so in the global cultural context of – and in reaction to – scientism, another fundamentalism whose faith is in the literal possibility of the omniscience and omni-competence of science. For these faiths, metaphor and analogy are not enough, nor is the vagueness of the eternal contemplation of the deity. Rather, the reward of the afterlife will be understandable in the terms of this life – as sensual pleasures, reunion with loved ones and so on. In the faith of scientism the completion of the scientific project would also involve a complete solution to the problems attendant on being human.

The pursuit of medical immortality is, in this context, evidently fundamentalist. It involves a literal extension of the experiences of this life. It is also scientistic in that it is based on a faith that it can be achieved, there can be no inherent logical barrier to our discovery of the means to sustain the human body forever. Curiously, however, the problems of what would be a virtual eternity on earth – boredom, repetition, the endurance of memory and attachment – have inspired many contemporary immortalists to move towards a scholarly or even Thomist conception of consciousness in the medically extended earthly paradise. The tension between the two eternities defined in Christian theologies persists in the philosophies of immortalism. Some say we can simply carry on as we are, the world is sufficiently varied and there is enough to learn and experience to sustain us through the centuries. Others say we will have to change ourselves – by, for example, medically expanding our brains – in order to avoid boredom and satiation. The conception of heaven continues to define the human imagination.

Various Fixes

Hermes Trismegistus (the thrice-greatest) was, for centuries, credited with producing the vast body of work known as hermetic literature. The word 'hermetic' – meaning obscure, hidden or belonging to the tradition of alchemy or magic – is derived from his name. He was the greatest sorcerer that ever lived and the creator of alchemy. Among Sir Isaac Newton's alchemical papers was found his own translation of Hermes's Emerald Tablet, fourteen sentences which contain the sum of all wisdom. Crucially –

> That wch is below is like that wch is above & that wch is above is like yt wch is below to do ye miracles of one only thing.
> And as all things have been & arose from one by ye mediation of one: so all things have their birth from this one thing by adaptation.

Hermes knew everything. He knew that everything was one and that everything could be transformed into everything else. The world was a single idea of a single mind.

Hermes stalks human history; he is everywhere. The words 'great, great, great' on the Rosetta Stone may refer to his triple greatness. He unified the two foundational civilisations of the West by combining the attributes of the Egyptian god Thoth – wisdom, magic – and the Greek god Hermes – the clever messenger, fleet of foot and full of trickery. Both these gods are psychopomps, guides to souls in the afterlife. The shadow of Hermes falls over medieval and Renaissance magic and, through Newton, over modern science. He embodies two enduring human convictions: that there is a secret wisdom that explains all things and that, beneath their surface disparities, all things are one.

It is, in this context, almost too banal to point out the obvious – that Hermes probably did not exist, that the writings accredited to him were produced by many authors over many centuries – because, imaginatively, he did, does and will continue to symbolise an ineradicable way of seeing the world. Hermes would not have been – is? – not astounded by quantum theory because he knew that our quotidian, common-sense view of the world concealed reality from our gaze. He would have regarded the insights of modern physics – that, for example, all matter is made from the same fundamental particles – as too obvious to be worthy of note. And he would definitely not have been surprised by our conviction that, through the application of our magic, we could conquer death. In the Emerald Tablet, he told us that there were means whereby we should 'have all ye glory of ye whole world & thereby all obscurity shall fly from you'. Men could become gods if only they knew.

Hermes Trismegistus is thus the true presiding deity of the pursuit of medical immortality. He represents the conviction that death can be conquered here on earth rather than in the hereafter. Before the age of science, it was always to his wisdom that aspirant immortalists deferred. He represents all previous attempts to find the technical fix that would prolong human life.

These attempts have been many, varied and frequently eccentric. None seem to have worked and all are regarded as little more than historical curiosities by contemporary scientists. Nevertheless, the forms of thought involved and the very fact that such attempts were made are both significant. Most significant may be the fact that previous techniques of prolonging life often look remarkably similar to the ones in which we now put so much faith.

Take the Taoists. Taoism can be read either as a philosophy or a religion, its central themes were laid down in works produced in China between 350 and 250 BC, most famously the Tao-te-Ching of Lao-tzu. Like Hermes, Lao may have had the good sense not to exist but, again like Hermes, he has exerted and continues to exert immense influence. There is one further similarity that hinges on the exact meaning of the word 'Tao'. Literally translated as 'The Way', it can also be taken to mean nature. More generally, it signifies the workings of the universe. To be at one with the Tao is to be at one with the underlying reality of the cosmos. This oneness represents a spiritual but also an ethical totality. To the true follower of the Tao, moral injunctions are meaningless, he just behaves righteously because he is at one with the way of things. That there is a way of things, an underlying reality, a unity, is implicit in hermeticism and, for that matter, contemporary physics.

In the original classics of Taoism, the attainment of oneness with this natural unity may have been a poetic or spiritual aspiration, a matter of contemplation rather than experiment. It was, however, subsequently interpreted as a practical matter. Through the disciplined pursuit of The Way, it was thought that life could be extended, perhaps indefinitely.

The techniques involved sound remarkably familiar. The Taoist conception of *wu wei* – effortless action – demanded calm and the avoidance of excess. Too much purposefulness was to be avoided and the correct political posture was quietism. Breathing exercises, gymnastics and frugal dietary habits were also recommended. The Taoists believed in the cultivation of the simple life. In short, they advocated the avoidance of stress, exercise, dieting and, had they had the choice, they would have eaten organic foods.

As in hermeticism, the idea of The Way implied a unity and interchangeability in all things. There was no sharp dividing line between things in nature, they flowed together. So the great Taoist alchemist Ko Hung said it was possible for animals to be changed from one species into another, for lead to be transformed into gold and for a human to be reconstituted as a *hsien*, an immortal being. Secret or lost techniques were involved which, it was believed, the greatest Taoist adepts had uncovered.

A number of important themes are embodied in Taoist thought. First, there is the idea that we are born with a quantity of life force which should not be expended by excess of any kind. The second theme is the Taoist conviction that the secrets of longevity or immortality had been known in the past. This was plainly a way of linking Taoist thought to older Chinese religious traditions, but such antediluvian myths about immortality are more or less universal. Most cultures have stories of ancient times when people lived to great ages. The Old Testament stories of the Bible are full of characters living for hundreds of years. In our time, it tends to be linked with a cult of primitivism. Modern myths include stories of people in distant lands who, untroubled by the stresses and pollutions of contemporary life, live to great ages. Yoghurt crops up frequently in these myths.

Antediluvian myths of immortality in distant times or hyperborean myths of immortality in distant lands both suggest there is a technical fix available to us in this life which has been lost but which can be found. Equally, the yoghurt suggests a third aspect of the mythology – the possibility of some material substance which can grant us longer life or, more commonly, actual immortality. This is usually seen as a special kind of water, as in the large number of fountain of youth myths. Most famously, in America at least, is the story of Juan Ponce de León, a Spanish conquistador who accompanied Columbus on his second voyage to the New World. Legend has it – and it seems to be nothing more than legend – that, once across the Atlantic, Ponce de León set out to discover either the fountain of youth or the River Jordan that was said to flow out of Eden through the newly discovered 'Indies'. In the event, he discovered Florida and thus became the first European known since the Vikings to have stepped on continental North America. Florida, in many different ways, remains in thrall to its foundational myth, the fountain of youth.

The persistence of such ideas through time can easily be demonstrated. The Epic of Gilgamesh, written on clay tablets dating back to 650 BC but probably based on a Sumerian story of 3000 BC, is a long poem about an arrogant young king, Gilgamesh, whom the gods try to subdue by creating a warrior, Enkidu. They fight but, subsequently, become close friends. Yet, ultimately, the gods kill Enkidu. Heartbroken, Gilgamesh confronts the possibility of his own death and sets off to discover the secret of immortality. The first secret offered to him is the austere, Taoist-like injunction to stay awake for six days and seven nights. Gilgamesh fails. The next idea is a plant which grows at the bottom of the sea.

Gilgamesh finds the plant, but it is eaten by a snake while he is bathing. The snake thus acquires the immortality denied to Gilgamesh. The story includes the hermetic, hyperborean and antediluvian myths – secret knowledge, distant lands and ancient times – as well as the self-discipline idea – the denial of sleep – and the immortalising substance – the undersea plant. All of these mythologies are still with us.

But the most important theme is that of the unity of all things, as manifested in the Taoist and hermetic traditions. This is important because it leads directly to our present pursuit of medical immortality. The connection is alchemy.

Alchemy is the golden thread or, rather, web that joins almost all aspects of human wisdom, the most advanced contemporary science included. Its origins are profoundly obscure both in space and time as it seems to have appeared in almost every part of the world in one form or another. The common themes are a concealed wisdom about the unity of all things and the interchangeability of all phenomena. The Western alchemical tradition is usually said to start with the Egyptians. The word itself is said by some to derive from the *Khem*, meaning the country of dark soil or Egypt. Others say it is derived from the Greek word *chumeia* which means casting or pouring together. Nevertheless, the most orthodox view is that the origins of alchemy lie in Egyptian metallurgy and it was the transmutation of metals that has always formed the core of alchemical wisdom.

A full history and summary of alchemy is probably beyond the intellect of any one man. It is fantastically complex, deeply mysterious and extraordinarily pervasive. But, for my purposes, the important alchemical theme is its close relationship to conceptions of and pursuit of immortality.

If the Egyptians provided the first practical demonstrations of alchemical processes through their metallurgy, it was the Greeks who provided the theory in the form of the idea of the four elements – earth, air, fire and water – and their inter-convertibility. This was to inspire the idea of the fifth element, the quintessence, the purified substance of which the non-earthly cosmos was formed. The Greeks also gave to alchemy the hylozoistic conception of the cosmos, the idea that all nature is alive and sentient, as well as the idea of a close link between the macrocosm and the microcosm, the link cele-brated in the words of Hermes Trismegistus – 'That wch is below is like that wch is above & that wch is above . . .'

But it was Plato who, in a crucial passage in the *Timaeus*, laid the foundations of the central idea of transmutability:

> In the first place, we see that what we now just called water, by condensation, I suppose, becomes stone and earth, and this same element, when melted and dispersed, passes into vapour and air. Air, again, when inflamed, becomes fire, and, again, fire, when condensed and extin-guished, passes once more into the form of air, and once more, air, when collected and condensed, produces cloud and mist – and from these, when still more compressed, comes flowing water, and from water comes earth and stones once more – and thus generation appears to be transmitted from one to the other in a circle. Thus, then, as the several elements never present themselves in the same form, how can anyone have the assurance to assert posi-tively that any of them, whatever it may be, is one thing rather than another?

This vision of a constantly flowing system in which one thing becomes another so seamlessly that the divisions cannot be seen is as much the vision of modern physics as it is of Taoism and of alchemy through the ages. Behind it lie the twinned ideas of oneness and perfectibility, ideas that were destined, for good or ill, to dog the Western mind.

The alchemy familiar to the popular imagination is the transmutation of base metals into gold deploying the catalytic effects of the philosopher's stone. Perhaps less familiar is the idea that this stone was also said to rejuvenate the human body and potentially confer immortality. Both ideas relate to perfectibility in that gold was regarded as the purest substance and immortality the idealised condition of man.

Via Arab thinkers like Khalid ibn Yazid, Jabir ibn Hayyan and Ibn Sinna (Avicenna) in the first millennium AD, alchemy was passed down to great Western adepts like Albertus Magnus, Roger Bacon, Paracelsus and the two great scientist-alchemists, Robert Boyle and Isaac Newton. Through this tradition, we can see alchemy gradually changing itself into modern science, though without losing its central conceptions of oneness and perfection.

In Isaac Newton the old wisdom and the new came together. He was both the last great sorcerer and the second – after Galileo – great modern scientist. In his commentary on the Emerald Tablet of Hermes, he wrote:

> Thus it ought first to be cleansed by separating the elements sweetly and gradually, without violence, and by making the whole material ascend into heaven through sublimation and then through a reiteration of the sublimation making it descend into earth: by that method it acquires the penetrating force of spirit and the fixed force of body. Thus will you have the glory of the whole world and all obscurities and all need and grief will flee from you. For this thing, when it has through solution and congelation ascended into heaven and descended into earth, becomes the strongest of all things.

After Newton, alchemy gave way to science. Its major themes remained intact. The current pursuit of the theory of everything in physics, for example, has obvious parallels with the concepts of oneness and purity in alchemy as well as the idea that all things, ultimately, are the same. But one theme was lost – the pursuit of immortality. This seemed beyond the reach of science here on earth and, meanwhile, that same science was undermining the foundations of belief in another, immortal realm. One way or another, the modern age had become an assertion of the finality of death. A backlash was inevitable, a backlash that attempted to turn the weapons of science against itself.

5

Hunting the White Crow

The Scole Group

Some years ago I wrote a story for the *Sunday Times* magazine about the Scole Group. Scole is a village in Norfolk. It was there that the group held regular seances. These had become world famous in spiritualist circles. In particular, they had become known for their use of 'physical mediumship'. This involves not just messages from another person in the spirit world, but actual physical manifestations. Their first success occurred on 4 October 1993 when an old coin – a Churchill crown – fell on to the table in the blacked-out basement room where three of the group were sitting. Such an object is known as an 'apport', meaning that it was a transfer of a physical object from one realm to another. This is a highly unfashionable approach. Physical mediumship, involving the familiar paraphernalia of psychokinesis, ectoplasm, spirit photography and apports, was a Victorian speciality. Like many such specialities, it had taken on a somewhat fusty, ridiculous air. Virtually all physical mediums are thought to have been unmasked as frauds. As a result, the very idea had been discredited. The spiritualism that flourished in the atmosphere of mass grieving that followed the First World War was almost entirely mental; people simply wanted to be in touch with their lost young men. Yet the Scole Group seemed to have resurrected the art of the physical mediums. Subsequent to the Churchill crown, the group was responsible for many more apports and for some spectacular and, even to sceptical observers, inexplicable effects.

I became involved because investigators from the Society for Psychical Research in London had produced a 100,000-word report on the group concluding that the phenomena were genuine and that evidence of human survival after death had been found. Investigations started in January 1995 and the report took three years to produce. The convinced investigators were planning an exhibition in London and they were hoping the *Sunday Times* would act as sponsor.

Journalism and spiritualism have long been natural companions. Newspapers can both report the sensational claims of spiritualists as if they were true and then take delight in exposing fraud when they find it. W.T. Stead, inventor of the now pervasive journalistic form of the interview, was one of the leading spiritualist advocates in the 1890s. Indeed, his list of interviewees extended beyond the living to include the dead. He also appears to have foreseen his own death. He once compared his role as prophet of the truths of the spirit world to a sceptical public to that of a drowning man. He died as a passenger on the *Titanic*.

Perhaps subliminally aware of this distinguished tradition, I took on the Scole story with an open mind. I had been commissioned without a hint of scepticism from the magazine's then deputy editor. Having no idea what people in general thought about the claims of spiritualists, I assumed that this was because she too had no set views on the subject. Though I did not think about it much, I considered it not absolutely inconceivable that the paper would, finally, back the exhibition. I seem to have been suffering from temporary insanity.

My open-mindedness was not based on careful assessment of the evidence but on a generalised sense that so many people had experienced so many things that there must be something in it. I had known highly intelligent people – my philosopher cousin Barrie, the writer Peter Ackroyd and many others – who had felt the same thing. I also had a more specific sense, since my childhood, that the world was full of inexplicable things. And I experienced a series of bizarre occurrences around the time of the birth of my daughter. We had moved into a new house and were effectively driven out of it less than a year later. There were countless accidents and misfortunes, all associated with the fabric of the house. The nastiest was when I tripped over a step, smashed my head into a cooker and came to halfway up the stairs covered in blood. The most suggestive involved doors flung open and sounds of voices from empty rooms. Several people, unprompted by us, said there was something wrong with the place. I remember one friend shuddering the moment he walked through the front door. A babysitter heard such dreadful noises that she had to turn up the television to drown them out.

When we sold the house – mentioning none of this to the snappy, aggressively business-like accountant who bought the place – a mournful neighbour with a comedy horror-film face came round to say, 'I didn't tell you before but that's always been an unlucky house.' Seemingly people had been watching us to see how we would cope with the spirits that infested the place. However, I drew no conclusions from this, seeing it as a purely practical matter. We just had to get out and, when we did, our lives returned to normal. The snappy accountant, I later learned, also sold soon afterwards.

But I had never been interested in spiritualism as such. It had seemed to me to be a shabby affair, partly because of the trickery and deception so often involved but mainly because of the sheer banality of the reported results. Messages from the spirit world seldom rose much above the level of a Hallmark card motto and never gave any evidence of any wisdom we could not attain unaided in this world. The Scole apports, meanwhile, were as gravely disappointing as any from past physical mediumship groups in that not one of them was an object that could not have been found in this realm. If the spirits were trying to prove something, they were failing miserably.

Nevertheless, I was welcomed into the Scole story with open arms.

'We are delighted you are doing this,' said Montague Keen, one of the Society for Psychical Research investigators, 'as the leading journalist in this field.'

Since, at the time, I had never written anything about spiritualism or any even remotely related topics, this was odd. Plainly, Keen was expecting a sympathetic article. Somewhat later, I discovered that the *Sunday Times* was expecting the opposite. They were expecting me to mock the Scole Group and, at one point, had grown concerned that I seemed to be on the verge of believing in the reality of what they took to be a lot of nonsense.

In the event, they were disappointed when my article – a judicious account of the evidence, concluding that nothing of any great significance had happened at Scole – turned out not to be a wildly comic account of gullibility and/or fraud. The problem was that I didn't find Scole funny, I found it sad.

Predictably, the story began to fall apart almost at once. Having read the SPR report – full of strange events but also full of holes – I asked to sit in on a seance. I could not because they had been discontinued after instructions from 'the other side'. I was, however, shown some videos of the other world, a set of colourful abstract shapes that had, it was said, appeared on the tape after the camera had been left in the dark in the basement room. They were quite pretty but hardly conclusive.

Frustrated by the spirits' veto of my seance experience, I visited a medium to see if I could acquire any sense of what might be involved. She was a friendly, decorous and serious lady who had been suggested by the College of Psychic Studies. But, though she saw a crowd of seemingly benign spirits around me, nothing they said made any sense at all. She did mention a philosopher and, since my cousin Barrie had just died, I reacted. But the spirit then delivered messages of such banality – 'stick to what you believe in' – that they could not possibly have been from the cousin I had known. Either it was not my cousin or he had become spectacularly dull in the afterlife. For aesthetic if not strictly scientific reasons, I preferred the former explanation. I received a wounded and amazed phone call from the college when I reported all of this in my article. They could not, it seemed, imagine the possibility of such total failure.

Further alarms bells rang when, for no very good reason, two of the Scole Group asked me to give them pseudonyms in the article. I did not do so.

Then – the final nail in the coffin of *Sunday Times* sponsorship of the Scole findings – other, more sceptical members of the SPR contacted me. They explained ways in which the basement effects could have been achieved and pointing out that elementary precautions – like the searching of the group before they went into the basement – had not been carried out. Their research was thorough and their findings detailed and devastating.

The article appeared and had, as far as I know, absolutely no effect on the spiritualists' conviction that something enormously important happened at Scole. I became a hate figure in these circles and, because I mentioned the story of our haunted house, I also became even more of a figure of fun than I already was among the hard-headed, sceptical scientist types.

The experience did, however, continue to, as it were, haunt me. First, I was left with an awareness of how amazing the experiences were in that basement room. Sceptics who had attended seances admitted the effects were astonishing and they had no idea how they were achieved. The SPR sceptics came up with a number of possible methods, but it was clear that the actual experience of being in that blacked-out room amidst apports, lights and countless other manifestations was highly persuasive.

Secondly, I was struck with the fervency of the will to believe. Many people involved were convinced beyond all possibility of refutation. Two of the SPR investigators, Keen and a retired electrical engineer named Arthur Ellison, both now dead, were remarkable for their absolute conviction that, whatever the banality of the spirit messages and the apports, whatever evidence was presented to show that some trickery was involved, some contact with the afterlife had been achieved at Scole. When I mentioned my banality problem to Ellison over lunch at his club, the Athenaeum, he simply agreed that it was a problem but didn't think it mattered. I was amazed at his insouciance. To me, the banality was crucial.

In the end, their belief seemed to come down to a rather stronger version of my own before I embarked on this story. I thought, weakly, that so many things seemed to have happened to so many people that something must be going on. They thought the same thing but much more strongly. They had the added conviction that spirit contact was actually the more likely explanation than fraud simply because the phenomena were so potent. In effect, they were appealing to the philosopher David Hume's warning about evidence of miracles.

'No testimony is sufficient to establish a miracle', he wrote, 'unless the testimony be of such a kind, that its falsehood would be more miraculous than the fact, which it endeavours to establish.'

But Hume was no believer in miracles. To him, this evidential test was insurmountable; there would *always* be less miraculous evidence of falsehood.

Thirdly, and most importantly, I was made aware of the oddity of the spiritualist project. What they are trying to do is find physical evidence in this world of immortality in another. In a fully religious context, this might not be so odd. In the Christian Middle Ages in Europe, for example, it would have seemed obvious that the physical facts of this world and the entire organisation of the cosmos provided evidence of God, heaven and hell. But the point then was that one would not have to look for such evidence. Reality itself was the evidence.

To the spiritualist, however, the evidence is concealed. The spirits may want to contact us and we them, but there are enormous obstacles. These might be obstacles that were intrinsic to the project, as seemed to be the case at Scole, or they might be obstacles in our mind. Throughout the history of spiritualism, mediums have complained that one sceptic in a room can ruin an entire seance. You had to believe to see the evidence. Sceptics laugh at this, saying it is evidence that the whole thing is a charade at the expense of the gullible. This may well be the case, but it may also be true that spiritualist or any extra-sensory power we possess are not like sight or hearing but like sexual arousal in the sense that they are dependent on context.

Concealment and obstacles are the clues to the central truth of spiritualism. It began as and still remains a project to reveal something – an ancient and natural human contact with the spirit world – that has either been lost or denied us by modernity. Modern science, since the early seventeenth century, had progressively been disenchanting the world, turning medieval 'reality' into modern reality. Far from revealing more of the truth, it had, in fact, succeeded in revealing less. For spiritualists, the spirits and the afterlife are scientifically real. Their existence can be proved or disproved. They are not a matter of faith. Spiritualism is thus an expression of the conviction that modern science has missed something – the final and irrefutable proof of our immortality.

'Faith', wrote Miguel de Unamuno, 'feels itself secure neither with universal consent, nor with tradition, nor with authority. It seeks the support of its enemy, reason.'

But, of course, in doing so, it separates itself from religion as traditionally understood. If there is proof, there is no need for faith and, therefore, no need for religion. And, indeed, many have pointed out that spiritualism is, in fact, inimical to religion.

'It must be clearly understood', observed C.S. Lewis, 'that if the Psychical Researchers succeeded in proving "survival" and showed that the Resurrection was an instance of it, they would not be supporting the Christian faith but refuting it.'

Spiritualism, as well as sundry other disciplines that I shall describe later, is an attempt to defend the existence of another realm from the onslaught of science. But, paradoxically, it is an attempt to do so that involves the application of the methods of science. The story of spiritualism is thus the story of an attempt to dispel the need for faith by the application of reason, an attempt that has been made many times before but never with such bizarre consequences. It is an attempt that is being made again in our time by the immortalists.

The White Crow

William James, brother of the novelist Henry, was a psychologist and philosopher. I have, humbly, always felt an affinity with the man. He was the creator of the philosophy of pragmatism, an attempt to view the world clear-sightedly without prejudgement, prejudice, preconceptions and, above all, without premature commitment. He was fragile, socially insecure and he could never make up his mind.

Intellectually, he was always on the edge of things, hovering indecisively over the frontier between the real and the imagined. He remains one of the greatest and most underrated figures of the modern age, a man whose imagination leapt beyond modernism to the postmodern quandary in which we now find ourselves. James, in the words of one admirer, 'defended the right to believe before all the evidence was in'. The eternal deferral of truth required by the patient investigations of science were too much for one lifetime. James wanted answers, but, on the other hand, he didn't.

Born in 1842 and dying in 1910, James lived through the great imaginative and religious crises which forged twentieth-century modernity. Above all, he saw the triumphs of geology and biology that seemed to crush forever the material foundations of faith. But, uncertain as he was, he could never quite bring himself to accept the imminent completion of the programme of Victorian materialism.

Yet he saw the problem clearly enough. The success of nineteenth-century science implied that everything, the human mind included, would one day be explained away, be drawn into the same materialistic fold as steam engines and monkey ancestors.

'How can we believe in life hereafter', he asked in *Human Immortality*: *Two Supposed Objections to the Doctrine*, 'when Science has once and for all attained to proving, beyond possibility of escape, that our inner life is a function of that famous material, the so-called "gray matter" of our cerebral convolutions? How can the function possibly persist after its organ had undergone decay?'

His answer was that the brain might not be the producer of thought, it may be the medium through which thought passed. Further, our biological state might, in fact, not be the precondition of thought but rather restrictive of its full expression. Released from its restraints, we might find ourselves floating free among our fellow spirits. He wrote: 'Suppose, for example, that the whole universe of material things – the furniture of earth and choir of heaven – should turn out to be mere surface-veil of phenomena, hiding and keeping back the world of genuine realities.'

This is not an anti-scientific idea. James was speculating about something that might be a fact in the world that had not yet been seen by the eyes of science. Once seen, there was no reason why this fact could not be incorporated into the body of scientific knowledge. And, as far as James was concerned, there was plenty of apparent evidence in the form of the colossal number of reports of contact with spirits that circulated throughout the Victorian and Edwardian eras.

Of course, a great many of these reports had turned out to be based on fraud. But, typically, pragmatically, James saw the true logic of the situation. The hardened sceptic might argue that if 99 per cent of reports of spirit contact were fraudulent, then it was reasonable to assume the remaining 1 per cent could be discounted. Either the fraud had not been detected or some error was involved. The sceptic might also add that the scientific method demands repeatability. The same results should follow from the same initial conditions. This did not seem to be the case with spirit contact; wildly differing results sprang from identical initial conditions.

But James turned the logic round. You do not disprove that all crows are black by examining every crow in the world to determine if it is black, you simply set out to find a white crow. One white crow would overturn the hitherto impregnable black crow hypothesis. Similarly one spirit contact would, if found to be genuine, be all that was required to topple the entire sceptic case. After all, the apple has only to fall upward once to topple Newton. I can imagine the excitement James must have felt at this possibility. At a stroke, it removed the need to plough through all the cases of fraud. All that was required was one case that was not fraudulent, one genuine contact, one white crow. In Mrs Leonora Piper, James found his white crow, his upward falling apple.

Strange Rapping Noises

Spiritualists say there is something in us that survives death. This something may not necessarily be immortal, though it is generally assumed to be. This is quite unlike mainstream religious beliefs which have, on the whole, either not set much store by immortality or have insisted on a final state in which body and soul are reunited. The idea of the separable soul as the one and only subject and object of salvation is more a product of modernity than of ancient tradition. Certainly it was present in Plato but it did not take on the lineaments of orthodoxy until the seventeenth and eighteenth centuries.

The reason for this is obvious. From Copernicus and Galileo onwards, the authority of science had steadily spread outwards into the physical world. The insistence that the earth revolved round the sun contradicted the Ptolemaic cosmology that had been endorsed by St Thomas Aquinas, and the physics of Galileo were seen by the Church as threatening the dogma of the 'real presence' of Christ in the bread and wine of communion. Faith thus found itself beleaguered as its material foundations were progressively eroded by science.

The new emphasis on the soul, the inner essence of the individual, was an attempt to escape from this threat. The post-medieval worldview placed ever greater emphasis on the soul. There were attempts physically to locate the seat of the soul. Descartes, for example, said it resided in the pineal gland, a pea-sized object in the brain, which, we now know, secretes melatonin, but whose function in the seventeenth century was entirely mysterious. But, increasingly, the soul was specifically defined as lying outside of our normal perceptions. Furthermore, this impalpable entity had become the authentic, the whole person, had invaded, as Aries puts it, 'every dimension of the individual'. The body became, in this soul-centred view, an irrelevance. By the nineteenth century the conviction of the absolute separability of soul and body was widespread. Unfortunately, its function – as a fortress against scientific explanation – could not easily be maintained. Something had to be done.

On 12 April 1848 in Arcadia, New York, one William Duesler gave birth to spiritualism when he wrote down his experiences in the house of his neighbours, the Foxes. Strange rapping noises had been heard, associated with the two Fox children, Katherine, eleven, and Margaretta, twelve. Duesler heard these rappings and, on the basis that the sounds were made by an intelligent, discarnate being, questioned the rapper. It gave answers, via raps, of unerring accuracy about such matters as the ages of Duesler and his wife. Many years later, the two children were to admit to perpetrating a trick – fraud at this stage would be much too strong a word –

involving beating on the floor with their toes; but, at the time, the news of what appeared to be genuine spirit manifestations spread rapidly. Indeed, even much later, when the fraud was admitted, convinced spiritualists remained unshaken in their convictions that the Fox sisters had contact with the next world.

The story of what followed has been told, with varying degrees of scepticism, elsewhere – notably by Ruth Brandon and Janet Oppenheim – so here I shall just focus on crucial features, all of them pointing to the central obsession with science.

The first point to make is that the spiritualist wave had some similarities to the UFO and alien abduction 'flap' that gripped first the US and then the world from 1947 onwards. Both had two distinct phases. Alien lore was first based simply on UFO sightings, but then, from the late sixties onwards, it became centred around accounts of alien abductions. It moved from vagueness to great particularity. The same thing happened with spiritualism. At first simply mental communication was involved, but later ectoplasm, spirit faces and figures as well as a variety of other physical phenomena manifested themselves. Again, there was a move to greater particularity. Both aliens and spirits became routine aspects of the popular imagination. By the late nineteenth century, seances were common occurrences in middle-class homes on both sides of the Atlantic and effective mediums were local celebrities. Alien invasion, meanwhile, became one of the standard plots of the era of movies and television. Both thrived in a climate of paranoia. Ufologists and spiritualists believed they were on to something that had either been deliberately concealed or simply missed by the authorities of the time, something of world-transforming value. They defined themselves as outsiders, truth-tellers from beyond the oppressive mechanisms of the age. Both were in rebellion against the apparent finality of science, its monopoly of wisdom and its vision of the universe as a cold and uncaring place. And yet both aspired to the condition of science.

The second point is that spiritualism also has similarities with the health and pro-longevity movements that blossomed from the late seventies onwards. The primary similarities here lay in the anxiety provoked by the spectacle of ageing and death and in the way mutual support communities and institutions formed around both spiritualism and the pursuit of health and longevity. Spiritualist circles are the correlative of Weight Watchers and institutions like the Society for Psychical Research anticipate the Immortality Institute. In addition, both movements have a strong proactive element in defiance of the problem, death, which they attempt to confront.

All of these similarities indicate the way people have tried to draw the project of the conquest of death into the realm of mainstream science. This brings me to the third and most important point about spiritualism. Once it had escaped from the rather specialised confines of rural New York state, it immediately attracted the attention of highly gifted and intelligent people, many of them among the leading scientists of their day.

This is not to say that the American religious climate in 1848 had nothing to do with the success of the Fox sisters. As the sisters' contemporary Alexis de Tocqueville pointed out, 'There is no country in the world where the Christian religion retains greater influence over the souls of men than in America.' It is an observation that remains true to this day. Furthermore, New England had been the birthplace of the Second Great Awakening, a sudden outburst of religious fervour, that swept the country from about 1800 onwards. Between 1776 and 1845, the number of preachers per capita in America tripled.

But there seems to have been a new literalness about these religious aspirations, a desire to find new forms of support for the faith. For example, hypnotism, then known as 'animal magnetism' or mesmerism after its discoverer Anton Mesmer (1734–1815), was interpreted as evidence of an unseen world. Specifically, a book by a preacher named George Bush entitled *Mesmer and Swedenborg* linked animal magnetism to the heavenly visions of the great Swedish mystic Emanuel Swedenborg. Spiritualism was part of the same pattern of seeking hard, observable evidence for faith. It was this that took spiritualism beyond America to Britain where, eleven years after the incidents at Arcadia, Darwin was to strike the deadliest blow of all against the unseen world with the publication of *On the Origin of Species*.

William Crookes, elected to the Royal Society after his discovery of the element thallium and unquestionably one of the most eminent scientists of the latter half of the nineteenth century, became interested in the physical medium Daniel Dunglas Home. Home was born in Edinburgh in 1833, though he first became a medium in America where he was brought up by an aunt. He returned to England in 1855 and became a celebrity, his seances being attended by the rich and famous. The poet Robert Browning was one, though unlike most he remained unconvinced and lampooned Home in his poem 'Sludge the Medium'. Nevertheless, Home remains perhaps the only physical medium whose reputation remains untainted by evidence of fraud. This is remarkable given that the effects he achieved seem to have been quite staggering. On 16 December 1868, for example, he was seen by apparently sane and sober observers to float out of one third-storey window and return through another. Ruth Brandon claims to find plenty of dubious elements in the reporting of this incident, but there is still no absolute evidence of fakery.

Crookes approached the phenomenon of spiritualism with

a high reputation for scientific objectivity, though Brandon feels this was compromised by the fact that he longed to believe in the reality of the phenomena following the death of his brother Philip in 1867 at the age of twenty-one. Nevertheless, the general conception that Crookes was an absolutely objective observer was decisive. His conviction that Home was genuine, that white crows were everywhere in Victorian England, effectively bestowed the blessing of hard science on spiritualism. With the founding of the Society for Psychical Research in 1882 and the further endorsements of eminent scientist Oliver Lodge, distinguished philosopher Henry Sidgwick, grand intellectual F.W.H. Myers and popular author Arthur Conan Doyle, it seemed that spiritualism had joined evolution by natural selection as one of the great discoveries of Victorian Britain.

Unfortunately all of these passionate, intelligent and frequently grieving people were repeatedly let down by the mediums themselves. Madame Blavatsky, mentor of among others W.B. Yeats, scarcely bothered to conceal her own fraudulence. Eusapia Palladino, once the great hope of the believers, was painfully obviously cheating – though this should not be taken as absolute proof of her fraudulence. The ghost photographs taken by the Nobel laureate physiologist Charles Richet and by the assiduous Baron von Schrenk-Notzing now appear – as they did to many at the time – ridiculously faked. Home excepted, all the physical mediums were seen to have been discredited by the less credulous SPR investigators. And so, by 1900, spiritualism was on the run.

Mrs Leonora Piper did much to reverse this sad decline in the seance business. She was born in New Hampshire in 1859. At the age of eight, while playing in the garden, she heard a voice whisper, 'Aunt Sara, not dead, but with you still.' She subsequently discovered that Aunt Sara had died at

that very moment. In 1884, she encountered a blind clair-
voyant, J.R. Cook, in whose presence she fell into a trance.
Later trances produced spirit messages of, it is said, remarkable accuracy.

Her reputation spread and finally, in 1885, William James
visited her at her Boston home. She impressed him with
knowledge of his family and of a recently deceased child, the
latter a very common spiritualist occurrence. After further
sessions, James became convinced of Piper's 'supernormal
powers'. She visited England in 1889 where even Frank
Podmore, the most ruthless exposer of frauds, was impressed
and accredited Piper with single-handedly reigniting enthusiasm for spiritualism.

Piper remains a presiding figure in spiritualism today, in
spite of the fact that in October 1901 she appears to have said
she had never been in contact with the spirit world. She did
not, like the Foxes, admit to cheating, but she did say that she
was inclined to accept a telepathic explanation of her powers.
James, asked to comment on the article in the *New York
Herald* in which this was reported, replied with typically sublime indecision that he was still 'sitting on the fence'.

It was Oliver Lodge who was to provide the most moving
affirmation of spiritualism. In September 1915, he lost his
beloved son Raymond, one more casualty of the Great War.
Via a strange message from Leonora Piper in August, Lodge
had seemed to have been given a warning of what was to
come. As soon as Raymond died, Lodge and his wife felt
they were in contact with him. His account of all the subsequent contacts with his son – entitled *Raymond* – was
published in 1916 and became the central text of the new
spiritualist wave that flowed in with the tide of grief felt by
millions in the aftermath of the trenches.

There Was No Message

James died of a heart condition in 1910. His brother Henry had travelled from England to Cambridge, Massachusetts, to be with him. Just before he died William asked Henry to stay on for six weeks. He said he would try to communicate from beyond the grave. That great novelist who, for the purposes of his work, heard everything, heard nothing from his brother, either because there was nothing to hear or because his ears had been stopped by the prejudices of his time. It is a pity. I should like to have heard more from William James. He would have been a more reliable reporter from the afterlife than any of the messengers at Scole.

What are We Human Beings, You and I?

The project to find a scientific basis for human survival after death continued, perhaps in slightly more muted terms, in the twentieth century. Previous failures and frauds, however, made the task ever more difficult. The competence of the fraudsters had been bewildering. Magicians and illusionists – notably the great and utterly indefatigable Houdini – proved to be more capable of seeing through their tricks than scientists. Furthermore, the alternative explanation for the mental phenomena – the explanation espoused, seemingly, by Mrs Piper – that mental mediumship was a telepathic effect, could not be ignored. The discovery of such a, as we would now call it, 'psi' effect would be a major breakthrough. It would amount to a triumphant demonstration that the world was not reducible to the terms of the more hard-headed, narrow-minded scientists. But it would not be evidence of immortality.

The most bewildering and complex attempt to overcome these difficulties was launched in 1901 by members of the

SPR. It was an experiment that was to run for thirty years. It was known as the Cross Correspondences. The basic idea was simple, the complexity arose in its application. The fundamental, as it were, atomic unit of mental mediumship was a message delivered to a medium who then reproduced it via speech or 'automatic' writing. Plainly any such message could be the result of cheating or telepathy. Delivering the same message through two mediums would reduce the likelihood of either, assuming the mediums had not been in contact. The next step is to deliver two different messages to the two mediums such that, individually, the messages would be incomplete or meaningless, but together would make sense. Extending this coding process to many mediums would, if successful, provide irrefutable evidence that the mediums were acting in exactly the way they said they were – as transmitters, not instigators, of the messages. On the other side of the equation, of course, it was necessary to have a dead person who knew the code. One was immediately to hand. Frederick Myers who died in 1901.

The vast documentation of the ensuing communications between Myers and multiple mediums is seen by believers as the most potent evidence in favour of survival. By sceptics, it is simply seen as another absurd concoction, riddled with wishful thinking and outright fraud. There seems to be evidence for both views. The correspondences do show remarkable expressions of classical learning known to Myers but probably not to all the mediums, as well as close links between the messages. Equally, there is evidence of complete confusion and failure.

I first heard of the Cross Correspondences when I visited Scole. Montague Keen assured me that he was convinced the evidence emerging from the Scole Group amounted to a continuation of the correspondences. The great Myers was still speaking from beyond the veil.

But, from the late 1920s onwards, the focus was to move from spiritualism to the more general concept of the paranormal. The great prophet of this change was Joseph Banks Rhine. Rhine, previously a botanist and plant physiologist, arrived at Duke University in North Carolina in 1927. There he was to establish the discipline of parapsychology and, in the words of the website www.rhine.org, naturalise 'the supernatural, bringing paranormal phenomena from the closed séance rooms of mediums into the open laboratories of experimental psychology'.

Like William James, though without the saving grace of genius, Rhine was mesmerised by how little, in spite of everything, we knew, specifically about the enigma of consciousness:

> What are we human beings, you and I? No one knows. A great deal is known about man, but his fundamental nature – what makes him behave as he does – is still a profound mystery. Science cannot explain what the human mind really is and how it works with the brain . . . No one even pretends to know how consciousness is produced. What kind of a natural phenomenon is thought? There isn't even a 'theory'. Such ignorance about the very knower himself is scarcely credible!

Starting from his (questionable) insistence that by 1930 the existence of the power of telepathy had been established beyond doubt, Rhine went on to say that: 'It looked as if the cerebrocentric hypothesis of man could not be maintained in face of the evidence for this extra-sensory mode of perception.'

In other words, the reductionist concept of thought as nothing more than an epiphenomenon of the workings of the brain could not be sustained. Nevertheless, Rhine was aware that the tide was running against any other interpretation, noting 'an unfortunate taboo . . . against discussion of the beliefs concerning man's ultimate nature'.

Rhine's work at Duke established to his own satisfaction the reality of a number of different psi capacities as well as telepathy – notably psychokinesis and clairvoyance. Unfortunately, few others were satisfied and a sad little note on rhine.org now informs us: 'Today, the Rhine Center is no longer associated with Duke, though it remains in Durham. Research methods have changed, but the research that J.B. Rhine initiated and did so much to promote continues in a new setting.'

The truth was that Rhine's results were far from indisputable and, more to the point, far from repeatable. Academic interest in the paranormal slumped disastrously after the brief flourishing under the influence of Duke. What interest remains seems to be largely anthropological or cultural. A somewhat forlorn summary of the position came to me in an e-mail from Dr Caroline Watt at the University of Edinburgh's Koestler Parapsychology Unit:

So far as I am aware, many of the existing attempts to investigate survival (in the form of seeing whether mediums are getting information about deceased persons represented by sitters) are methodologically flawed . . . and there has not yet in my opinion been any persuasive evidence for survival. 'Platform' mediums are very popular, but it appears that they are simply using psychological techniques such as cold and hot reading (as well as editing in the case of TV programmes) to give the appearance of giving information from a deceased person.

Of course, Rhine's work was not primarily about survival, but it shared with spiritualism this central conviction that science had either failed to take note of or was wilfully ignoring evidence from beyond its narrow worldview. Again, the aim was not to use religion as a stick with which to beat science, but rather to bring what was previously called religion into the realm of science. A minor but crucial theme in all this work is the conviction that, in fact, unaided by the spiritualists and the paranormalists, science and religion were converging of their own accord. It was the science of Mesmer that persuaded many of the truth of spiritualism, for example, and even the technology of Alexander Graham Bell inspired Oliver Lodge. Though science may have invaded the realm of magic and religion, technology seemed to show that the magic was really there. If voices could travel great distances down a telephone, perhaps they could also cross the barrier of death.

But there is a deep and unresolved contradiction here, captured in a remark by one of the most enthusiastic of spiritualists, Sir Arthur Conan Doyle: 'We want to get something that will beat materialism, we want a religion that you can prove.'

A religion that could be proved would be science and, therefore, merely an expanded materialism. The white crow would overturn the theory that all crows were black, but it would not establish the colour of all crows. Materialistic science would survive the shock of first contact with the spirit world. Indeed, it would thrive on the encounter.

It Scared the Shit Out of Me

There is, however, one crucial footnote to this story. Spiritualism survives today, but in specialised enclaves. Popular newspapers give it some credence and various mediums and spiritualistic institutions – one in Boston, the First Spiritual Temple, is devoted to the work of Mrs Piper –

continue to maintain their increasingly beleaguered faith. There is, plainly, still an immense popular appetite for this form of consolation. In Glasgow Gordon Smith, the psychic barber, is British spiritualism's pop star. His website boasts that the *Daily Mail* has said he is 'Hailed as the UK's Most Accurate Medium'. And I routinely have conversations with highly intelligent people who assume, in an unexamined way, that there must be 'something in it'. Nevertheless, the great wave of Victorian and Edwardian fascination with spiritualism has ebbed. It persists, for the majority, as a background superstition, as something entertaining, perhaps even thought-provoking, perhaps vaguely indicative that there are more things in heaven and earth, but not as something it is necessary or even socially acceptable to do anything about. Academically and scientifically, the whole business is regarded as being discredited, disproved and a laughable example of the inability of the human imagination to come to terms with our entirely material destiny. This is almost a universal consensus. But not quite.

Stephen E. Braude is Professor of Philosophy at the University of Maryland. He began his academic career as a distinguished but mainstream analytical philosopher. But, in doing so, he had effectively suppressed the memory of a childhood experience of a seance. A table moved and spelt out messages from a spirit called Horace T. Jecum.

'I was absolutely not prepared for this,' he told me, 'I was very much brought up into the standard materialistic, reductionist world view . . . It scared the shit out of me. I put it out of my mind. I was just interested in getting a job, I couldn't deal with it . . . Later, when I had the comfort of tenure, I realised, if I was honest, I needed to think about this. If I took my role as a philosopher seriously, then I needed to think about the implications of this.'

Braude was aware of the very respectable figures of the

past – among many others, James and the British philosopher C.D. Broad – who had studied spiritualist phenomena, but he also quickly became aware of the way the whole field had become academically toxic. Everybody assumed the story of spiritualism was simply a tale of the fraudulent and the gullible.

'In fact, to my surprise, I quickly realised that people didn't have a clue what they were talking about . . . It was a combination of embarrassment and intellectual dishonesty in many cases.'

Braude embarked on an examination of the evidence, at first mainly from physical mediumship. In *The Limits of Influence: Psychokinesis and the Philosophy of Science*, he went back to the great physical mediums and their debunkers and concluded that something we would now call 'paranormal' was indeed happening. In *Immortal Remains: The Evidence for Life After Death*, he went much further:

'And I think we can say, with little assurance but with some justification, that the evidence provides a reasonable basis for believing in personal postmortem survival. It doesn't clearly support the belief that everyone survives death; it more clearly supports the belief that some do. And it doesn't support the belief that we survive eternally; at best it justifies the belief that some individuals survive for a limited time.'

Braude's method is simply to look as clear-sightedly as possible at the evidence. In the case of Eusapia Palladino, for example, it is undeniable that she was often found to be cheating. But he makes the point that her cheating was obvious and crude. On other occasions, the phenomena were sufficiently convincing to baffle even the most sceptical observers. If she was bad at cheating, as she evidently was, then something else must have been happening when no cheating could be detected. One or more episodes of cheating should not, therefore, necessarily result in the dismissal of a medium's entire work. This is an important argument because of the general assumption among sceptics that fraud – and there was a very great deal – discredited the entire enterprise. In Braude's interpretation, successful mediumship was not discredited, merely camouflaged by fraud.

His other crucial argument is aimed at the discrediting of spiritualism by science. In spite of the best efforts of Rhine and others, it is clear that paranormal effects have proved unrepeatable in the laboratory. That, combined with the claim made by many mediums that the presence of sceptics can hamper the effectiveness of their powers, had seemed to confirm that the whole thing is some kind of trick or fix. But Braude argues that it is perfectly possible that mediumistic powers are similar to, say, sexual arousal rather than like sight or hearing. They are highly sensitive to context and more like an emotion than a sense. If so, then they may well lie beyond any possibility of conventional scientific analysis. This is not an especially exotic idea. We are currently a long way from analysing consciousness in terms of brain processes. It is therefore perfectly reasonable – indeed, it is obvious – to say that some human capacities lie beyond the competence of the laboratory. In addition, when science cannot explain a phenomenon, some degree of speculation is perfectly acceptable. Braude points out that physicists have posited the existence of so far unobservable 'dark matter' to explain the structure of the cosmos. Why then is it not legitimate to posit the soul as an explanation of certain human phenomena?

Under the Knife

Death, as I have said, has been redefined in our time. It is no longer the mere cessation of the heart, it is the death of the brain. Since the latter is less easily defined and since the brain can survive the cessation of the heart for a short period, we have created a period of uncertainty when we can't be sure of life or death. More resonantly we have created a period in which we – or rather our doctors or relatives – can decide whether we live or die.

There are numerous implications. We might, for example, conclude that death is a culturally arbitrary construct; it is merely the point at which the competence of current medical technology expires. Or we may be thrown into turbulent ethical debates about whether we can 'play God' by deciding whether brain-dead but not heart-stopped patients should live or die. Or, in the same context, we may wonder when the 'self' is no longer present in a body in such an ambiguous condition. Or we may decide that those who return from this no-man's-land between life and death have, in fact, returned from death itself and can report on what they saw.

This is the idea behind the contemporary fascination with Near Death Experience (NDE) and the closely associated Out of Body Experience (OBE). People who are brought back to life have, it is thought, literally been 'near' death; they have in some sense looked it in the face and had a glimpse of what lies beyond. Surveys have consistently shown that a significant minority – usually around 10 per cent – of people who have cardiac arrests have NDEs. Like spiritualism and the paranormal, this is a phenomenon that occurs alongside, not outside, science. In this case it is the development of medical technology that makes the experience possible or, at least, frequent enough for it to be observed. Yet, again like spiritualism and the paranormal, its relationship to science is ambivalent. Believers in the significance of NDEs say it shows the blindness or limitations of our scientific view while, at the same time, wishing their beliefs to be validated scientifically.

One aspect of NDEs, however, is seldom remarked upon. This is its theological ancestry. The Christian view of exactly what happens after death has changed radically over time. The dominant view until around the sixteenth and seventeenth centuries was that at death the individual went into a kind of sleep. On the Day of Judgement, he was awoken and judged. In some versions, only the saved are woken, the damned are simply left to oblivion. Either way, the point is that there is a period of suspension between death and judgement. This began to change when new players appeared in the depiction of deathbed scenes. These were the angels and demons that danced around the dying person's bed, seen by him but not by his relatives and friends. This marked the new idea that judgement took place at the moment of death rather than at some point in the distant future.

The notion of death as a decisive moment entered the vernacular, even of the secular world. At moments of great danger, people now routinely report that 'my whole life flashed before my eyes'. This 'life review' effect is plainly linked to the idea of instant judgement on death. The link between the biography and the moment of death has been deeply embedded in people's minds, death having become, almost literally, a mirror of the life. The importance attached to NDEs is an aspect of this popular view.

But, like many such phenomena, it seems to have an ancient ancestry. An academic, Sam Parnia, notes a passage in Plato's *Republic* where a soldier wounded in battle experiences a movement from darkness to light accompanied by angels, a passage through a tunnel to a bright light in the Hieronymous Bosch painting *The Ascent into the Empyrean* and the accounts of a nineteenth-century Swiss mountaineer of thirty accidents in which victims reported similar experiences. Parnia also points to NDE accounts with the same basic features from China, India and South America. Others have pointed out that the idea is present in the Old Testament, in *The Tibetan Book of the Dead*, a guide to how to conduct oneself in the period immediately after death, and in Swedenborg.

Near-death visions were first identified as a distinct phenomenon in our time when, in 1926, a psychical researcher and Fellow of the Royal Society, Sir William Barrett, published a book about visions seen by the dying. But this was at a time when people still died at home surrounded by friends and family. The reports of the dying were heard by others. Hospital deaths tend to suppress such visions either because they happen without company or because the patient is heavily drugged. On the other hand, modern technologies capable of bringing people back from the brink of death mean that people are able to report on the experience.

There was, in addition, one very prominent account given by the pyschologist Carl Gustav Jung. Jung had a heart attack in January 1944 and reported: 'What happens after death is so unspeakably glorious that our imagination and our feelings do not suffice to form even an approximate conception to it . . . The dissolution of our time-bound form in eternity brings no loss of meaning.'

NDEs have now become the subject of a movement whose adherents seem to be startlingly numerous. Two key figures were responsible for the popular dissemination of the idea. One was Raymond A. Moody, a medical doctor and philosopher, whose book *Life After Life* effectively launched the idea in the seventies. The other was Elisabeth Kübler-Ross, a psychiatrist and leading figure of the modern movement to provide counselling for the dying.

Moody's book, *Life After Life: The Investigation of a Phenomenon – the Survival of Bodily Death*, does not, he warns, aspire to prove life after death, such proof is not presently possible. Rather, it is simply about numerous reports from people who had almost died of certain highly specific experiences. These typically involve buzzing sounds, a tunnel down which the individual is walking, a bright light and, frequently, the impression of a border or boundary represented by a wall or fence. Moody is also anxious to establish that these experiences are timeless, rather than simply dependent on advances in medical technology. Throughout, he says, we find 'striking parallels' of contemporary accounts of NDEs.

Though Moody is relatively cautious about the ultimate significance of NDEs, his book is a clear assertion of the separability of body and soul, the same concept that drove spiritualism. Autoscopy – seeing one's own body from outside, the so-called out of body experience (OBE) – is, in this context, perhaps the most revealing aspect of the phenomenon. People frequently report looking down on themselves, typically on an operating table. The clear implication is that the soul has escaped from the body and beneath that is the assumption that the soul is the real and complete person.

(In fact, the 'core experience' of the NDE was best outlined by a study of 102 patients who had been near death at the University of Connecticut in 1980. Some 50 per cent experienced five distinct stages: peace, body separation, entering the darkness or tunnel, seeing the light and entering the light.)

Kübler-Ross, however, was a good deal less cautious than Moody. The bright light is the NDE that has most effectively penetrated the popular imagination. She, in her book *On Life After Death*, is quite clear about its meaning:

In this light, you will experience for the first time what man could have been. Here there is understanding without judging, and here you experience unconditional love. In this presence, which many people compare with Christ or God, with love or light, you will come to know that all your life on earth was nothing but a school that you had to go through in order to pass certain tests and learn special lessons.

She indicates that this experience of dying reveals the true nature of our earthly lives:

> It is an opportunity that you are given to grow. This is the sole purpose of existence on this planet earth. You will not grow if you sit in a beautiful flower garden and somebody brings you gorgeous food on a silver platter. But you will grow if you are sick, if you are in pain, if you experience losses, and if you do not put your head in the sand but take the pain and learn to accept it not as a curse, or a punishment, but as a gift to you with a very, very specific purpose.

And finally she concludes that death itself is an illusion and associates this discovery with contemporary conceptions of human guilt:

> But my *real* job is, and this is why I need your help, to tell people that death does not exist. It is very important that mankind knows this, for we are at the beginning of a very difficult time. Not only for this country, but for the whole planet earth. Because of our own destructiveness. Because of nuclear weapons. Because of our greediness and materialism. Because we are piggish in terms of ecology, because we have destroyed so many, many natural resources, and because we have lost all the genuine spirituality.

This is a familiar lament for the failings of our age. Here it is significant because it links our guilt with our mortality. Kübler-Ross suggests our inability to see our own immortality is the consequence of sin. This, of course, is one interpretation of the story of Genesis. Death was brought into the world when Adam and Eve ate the fruit of the tree of knowledge of good and evil. Our resulting exile from Eden was an exile into mortality from our natural condition of immortality – how, after all, could Eden have been paradise if it was tainted with the prospect of death?

Perhaps because of such deeply embedded associations, the NDE movement has succeeded in penetrating the popular imagination. The 1990 film *Flatliners*, mentioned earlier, takes the fact that there are such experiences as a given. It also follows Kübler-Ross in directly associating the moment of death with a drama of sin and redemption. The additional theme in the film is the technological competence of the young doctors. They are able to induce NDEs by subjecting themselves to what would once have been known as death, but which, in hospital conditions, becomes merely a hiatus in life. This is an odd device that could mean either that technology has found a way of cheating God by allowing us to see his designs through the pretence of death or that Kübler-Ross is right and that death is some kind of illusion, a product of our fallen condition.

It is clear from NDEs that medical technology gives an opportunity for the reassertion of some very ancient human intuitions, not least about guilt and redemption. It also offers new ways of expressing the conviction that there is within us a soul, an essence, which is separable from our bodies. Perhaps the point is that the ability of science to penetrate so far into our bodies convinces people that there must be a point at which this separable essence becomes apparent, as if by digging deep enough into the ground we must eventually find hell. Or alternatively we have found that this essence is, in fact, dispersed throughout the body.

There are, of course, somewhat less resonant scientific theories. The psychologist Susan Blackmore rightly dismisses the hard sceptical view that these phenomena are 'just

hallucinations'. To say this is to say nothing about such a pervasive and consistently reported phenomenon. Her own
tentative theory is that the tunnel experience may be related
to peculiarities in our visual field. OBEs, meanwhile, often
occur in people who are not near death but rather falling
asleep or suffering from migraine or epilepsy. At such
moments our methods of assessing what is real falter. In
normal consciousness, we are processing memories and associations as well as immediate perceptions, and this produces
multiple models from which the brain is programmed to
choose the best and most stable. If this process is disrupted,
we find ourselves adrift and, indeed, the life review may occur
because we are adrift in a memory model. Furthermore, the
OBE may occur because frequently these memory models
have been found to give the impression of seeing things from
an external viewpoint. At the furthest limits of the experience,
the profundity of the feelings associated with NDEs may be
explained by the complete dissolution of the self in this shifting realm. Dissolution of the self is, of course, an aspiration in
many religious practices.

The convergence of religion and science implicit in such
theories is important. Blackmore does not deliver the message
that the most fervent enthusiasts of NDEs and OBEs would
want to hear – that this is evidence of the existence of the soul
and of survival beyond death. But, crucially, she does take the
experiences seriously, she affirms their reality. Her explanation of what causes them is secondary and, anyway, does not
in itself disprove alternative theories. This could be what happens in the brain, but it could be the result of, rather than the
cause of, the phenomena. The story recapitulates that of spiritualism and shows again that evidence provided by science
has encouraged people to draw very different conclusions
from the scientists.

There is one further continuation of this story in our time.

The phantom limb phenomenon is well known. After an accident or an amputation, people frequently feel that the lost limb is still present – they feel itching or pain. This common but bizarre phenomenon can seem highly suggestive. Admiral Lord Nelson, for example, suffered twinges in the arm he had lost during the attack on Santa Cruz de Tenerife. He took these twinges to be evidence that we have incorporeal souls. His assumption was that our souls may be separable from our bodies, but they are not like Descartes's pineal gland, located in one small organ, rather they are coextensive with our material bodies, an idea expressed by Wittgenstein when he said the best picture of the human soul was the human body.

In our day we have organ transplants, a procedure that at least calls into question the idea of the coextensive soul. But it does not do so if you argue that, in receiving somebody else's heart or kidney, you are receiving some aspect of the donor. This is the argument of Claire Sylvia in her book *A Change of Heart*, the primary textbook of a small subculture of belief that transplanted organs do also result in partial soul transplants. Sylvia had a heart-and-lung transplant and began to take on some of the characteristics of the donor, like his love of beer, Snickers and green peppers. She also became more masculine. This all happened to her before she discovered who the donor was.

Always the constant theme is that mainstream science is barking up the wrong tree. It is missing big and highly suggestive phenomena. Indeed, it may be conceptually at fault. NDEs and OBEs, in particular, could be taken to imply that the neuro-scientific pursuit of the roots of consciousness in the material structure of the brain is entirely misconceived. Perhaps consciousness is irreducible in such terms, a force rather than a separable phenomenon. This is close to the speculations of William James. Or, as Roger Scruton has argued, the very idea of consciousness is simply not a scientific matter, it is philosophical. There is, in these terms, a limit to what can and cannot be said scientifically. Any limit, of course, requires something beyond.

The Black Crow

To repeat: all the travellers on the road from spiritualism to NDEs, phantom limbs and transplanted organs have been walking alongside science. These phenomena and projects have certainly been attempts to cope with the onslaught of scientific knowledge and the threat it seemed to pose to established religion, but also to the whole less well-defined penumbra of faith, intuition, belief and to the sense of the human self. These things are not called religion – though I think they are – but they are equally threatened by an imperious form of knowledge that aspires, one day, to explain all things through a single method, to see all things through the eyes of a single, material god. Something in people consistently rebels against this possibility and seeks succour in whatever consolations might be on offer, however bizarre.

The irony is, of course, that the consolations on offer are linked to scientific progress. Distinguished scientists gave spiritualism respectability, and science, through medical technology, has provided the opportunity for claims about NDEs and the transplantation of a personality with an organ. But now, if Stephen Braude is right, an orthodoxy of hard scientism has risen up to crush these evanescent insights and we are in danger of losing the opportunity to attain an understanding that would transform our sense of human destiny. We would have failed, in the words of Alan Gauld, one of the SPR investigators who first raised doubts about the Scole Group, 'to catch the biggest fish of all'.

Or rather, we would have missed another animal, the white

crow. That bird is, in the end, immortality or, in the terms of the spiritualist investigators, survival of the self through the ordeal of death. Both in the churches and in obscure corners of quasi-scientific belief, the faith lingers on that the soul is the only mechanism that can deliver survival. But out there among the new immortalists there is no need for any such obscure superstition. Soon we shall keep the body alive, so who needs a soul? The crows are all black and, what is more, they are on the wing.

6

Survival Now?

After Alchemy

Having been despatched by a magazine editor to the Clinique La Prairie in Montreux, I chose to decline the injections of foetal lamb cells. This may have been foolish. Charlie Chaplin, Marlene Dietrich and Pope Pius XII had all taken the course and, subsequently, enthused about the results. I dislike injections, however, and always feel uneasy in Switzerland.

Nevertheless, I had been intrigued to come in contact with the practical application of the theories of Paul Niehans. In the 1930s, Niehans, a Swiss doctor, pursued, initially, the cure of disease through the injection of young mammalian cells. Subsequently, the technique came to be seen as a method of rejuvenation. The idea was persuasive. The rich, the famous and the powerful bought the treatment. They still do so, as I observed at Montreux. La Prairie also offers a more conventional health regime of diet and exercise as well as cosmetic surgery. But the cell therapy – using unborn lamb's livers – made its name.

Mainstream science pours scorn on the idea.

'Personally,' writes British gerontologist Tom Kirkwood, 'there is no way I would ever let anybody inject sheep or goat cells into any part of my anatomy. Not only is there a risk of adverse immunological reaction, or of cross-species transmission of pathogens, but what good can it do? The immune system is designed to recognise and rapidly destroy foreign cells.'

The immune system, however, cannot destroy vanity and hope. And, in fairness to Chaplin and Dietrich, there is something very literal and understandable about the idea of being given young lamb cells to revitalise old human ones. It feels as though it just might work. And, as ever, what is the alternative?

Niehans's cell therapy was one among many attempts to find a scientific way to a longer life. After the decline of alchemy and the rise of the experimental method in the seventeenth century, it was natural to assume that the same technique could be applied to the human body. There was one immediate and spectacular success. In 1616, just seven years after Galileo had first looked through a telescope, the Englishman William Harvey announced his discovery of the circulation of the blood. This pump and pipe model of the body's systems was to be suggestively analogous to the machines of the next century's Industrial Revolution. The body, it seemed, was a machine that could be fixed and tinkered with. In the eighteenth century, this idea was further reinforced by Edward Jenner's discovery that cowpox could be used as an inoculation against the much deadlier disease of smallpox. The body was a smart machine, but now we could make it smarter. In the nineteenth century, Louis Pasteur's germ theory of disease dramatically affirmed the continuing success of science in uncovering the processes of the body and the identity of its enemies.

A parallel tradition was the scientific study of human longevity. There have always been stories of prodigiously long-lived people, one of the most celebrated in the age of science being Thomas Parr – 'Old Parr' – whose grave in Westminster Abbey suggests he died aged 152. On his death in 1635, William Harvey performed the autopsy on Parr. His apparent great age had made him a celebrity. Harvey could not ascertain Parr's true age, but did note that he was old and healthy but for the blood in his lungs that had, presumably, killed him. Research in the nineteenth century was to show that Parr's longevity was almost certainly a myth, probably propagated by Parr himself.

Confident Victorians were enthused by the idea that their burgeoning scientific competence could be applied to the apparently uncontrollable phenomenon of death. This enthusiasm was matched by an even more powerful horror at the stark facts of human dissolution. Two of the greatest writers of the age – Leo Tolstoy and Gustave Flaubert – produced books whose impact depends on their unblinking focus on the facts of our all too easily subverted physicality. Tolstoy's shattering novella *The Death of Ivan Ilyich* is simply the account of a man's death. But the very fact that he chose to write such an account is an indication that there was something new and terrible to be said. For death had, in Tolstoy's time, become incomprehensible in an entirely novel way. The *muzhiks* – the peasants – still seemed to die at peace; their death was expected and understood as an essential aspect of life. On his own deathbed, Tolstoy asked, 'What about the muzhiks? How do the muzhiks die?'

But bourgeois decency does not offer peace. Ilyich's death is dirty, disgusting and denied. The convention of lying to the patient had been born. But this was not just an aspect of decency, it was an aspect of medicalisation. Increasingly in the nineteenth century, the dying were attended by doctors who had to be seen to be doing things, in spite of the fact there was very little they could do. Ilyich's death is medicalised, denied and rejected. As a result, it becomes utterly incomprehensible:

> Another fortnight passed. Ivan Ilyich now no longer left his sofa. He would not lie in bed but lay on the sofa. And facing the wall most of the time he lay and in solitude suffered all the inexplicable agonies, and in solitude pondered always the same insoluble question: 'What is it? Can it be true that it is death?' And the inner voice answered: 'Yes, it is true.' – 'Why these agonies?' And the voice answered, 'For no reason – they just are so.' Beyond and besides this there was nothing.

Similarly, in Madame Bovary, Flaubert goes to gleeful lengths to describe in detail the death of his heroine from poisoning. Equally significantly, at the centre of the book there is the long account of a hideously botched operation on a man's foot. Both these writers were trying to present us with the unbearable spectacle of death stripped of all meaning and consolation. The even more savage twist is the incompetent medical procedures that accompany these deaths. For Flaubert and Tolstoy, the technology served only to heighten the agony.

Nevertheless, the scientific effort continued. Much work went into the study of how people died. However, as I have already mentioned, the crucial breakthrough was not medical but statistical. In 1825 Benjamin Gompertz discovered a remarkable consistency in death rates. The risk of death in adult humans doubles every eight years. A similar progression, though over shorter time periods, occurs in other animals. This insight was to provide the basis of the life

insurance industry and led directly to our current definition
of ageing as an increasing chance of dying.

In the twentieth century, medicine, combined with public
health measures, finally succeeded in producing the greatest
ever increase in human longevity. By attacking infectious diseases through better sanitation and, latterly, antibiotics and
inoculation, by improving nutrition and, probably most
important of all, through cutting infant mortality rates, science presented mankind with the gift of more life. Between
1900 and 2000, life expectancies at birth in the developed
world rose from the high forties to the mid to late seventies.
They have continued to rise, though nobody is quite sure
why. It was assumed the figures would hit a plateau. This
hasn't yet happened, possibly because of generally better
nutrition, health care and ways of life, involving more exercise and less smoking. Conservative estimates now suggest
that, even without any fundamental medical innovations, life
expectancies may rise into the nineties over the next century.
Given that prehistoric man is thought to have had a life
expectancy of about eighteen years, modern man is blessed
indeed, having sixty and possibly as many as eighty additional years.

He isn't grateful. Living longer has just made him more
anxious and demanding. In 1900 the major killers were infectious diseases, in 2000 they were heart disease, cancer and
cerebrovascular disease (stroke). This led to a widespread
conviction that diseases were, somehow, caused by modern
life. This is true but only because we live longer, not, primarily, because of what we do with our lives. Smoking certainly
has some effect on cancer rates – and on the incidence of
other lethal conditions – but almost all the other health scares
are either irrelevant or trivial in their impact.
Overwhelmingly, we get cancer because we breathe oxygen, a
highly toxic substance. Oxygen metabolism leads to the

production of free radicals, unstable compounds which strip electrons from neighbouring molecules, rendering them unstable. This chain reaction can lead to damage in the DNA. Normally, this is repaired and, even if it isn't, it may be harmless. In addition, free radicals only last for about a millionth of a second. Occasionally, however, a cancer suppressing gene may be knocked out. Cancer is clonal, it starts from a single cell. The damaged gene grows uncontrollably and, ultimately, forms a tumour. This is an improbable chain of events but it only needs to happen once and there are trillions of cells in the body. Statistically, therefore, it is very likely to happen over a long enough period of time. A third of us will contract cancer before we die. Cancer happens because we live long enough for it to happen. The same is true of most of the modern killers.

Oddly, however, even if we cured cancer tomorrow, the effect on longevity would be minimal. American gerontologist Leonard Hayflick calculates that a cure for cancer would increase life expectancy at birth by 3.1 years and by 1.9 years at the age of sixty-five. More sensational would be a cure for cardiovascular disease. That would add 13.9 years at birth and 14.3 years at sixty-five. Yet, even so, what is striking about these figures is how low they are. We fret and fuss endlessly about avoiding or curing these diseases, but even if we did, it seems, our lives would remain roughly as limited as they already are. Hayflick reckons that even if we cured all current causes of death, we would not increase life expectancies as much as we did in the twentieth century.

This strongly indicates that there is such a thing as a lifespan, a time limit beyond which the human body cannot go, even if disease free and sustained by the best possible environment with optimum nutrition. The best estimates for our lifespan are in the 115 to 120 range with Jean Louise

Calment's 122 years of life being the most anybody can hope for.

But there is something rather weird about this lifespan idea. After all, if the human body is a fixable machine, then the idea of a lifespan seems as magical or mysterious as a life force or a soul. We could talk of cars as having a lifespan, but it would be an arbitrary figure. We know we could conceivably make cars immortal just by continually replacing their parts. To suggest that we can't do the same for humans is to imply that there is something special about them. And that goes against the grain of everything we have discovered through science. The body is just organised matter. Therefore, it must be fixable.

This conviction became even stronger thanks to the twentieth-century's successes in increasing longevity. As a result, rather than sitting back and being grateful for the extra years, people sought ever more radical technological fixes. If I can live this long, why not longer? Furthermore, the twentieth century also introduced us to old age on an unprecedented scale. Both in ourselves and in others, we saw the ravages of time on the human frame. In the past, people had avoided seeing this spectacle in themselves or others by the simple expedient of dying. But now it was all around us and within us. Dying to avoid it was too much to ask and so we sought to defeat it.

From the late-nineteenth century onwards, new medical cures for ageing and dying were everywhere. Charles-Edouard Brown-Sequard ground up animal testicles and injected them into humans. Eugen Steinach grafted young men's testicles on to those of old men. Then there was the yoghurt theory, a hardy perennial. These were serious attempts, offered in all sincerity. There were also many hucksters in this business, however. Writing in the sixties, the historian of science Gerald J. Gruman noted wearily the unfortunate story of all these failed or fraudulent attempts: '. . . there are few subjects which have been more misleading to the uncritical and more profitable to the unscrupulous; the exploitation of this topic by the sensational press and by medical quacks and charlatans is well-known.'

What follows in this chapter is where we stand now in this story. In the simplest terms, we are still in the midst of that history of which Gruman, a keen immortalist, writes so despairingly. Hucksters still surround us, shouting their wares, whether they are cosmetics, 'alternative' treatments, dietary supplements or lifestyle changes. We are also daily assaulted by health scares – at the time of writing, the primary one is bird flu – and speculative journalism about cures for this or that. None or some of these things might be true. All cannot be. Here, however, is the story of what may or may not be the most viable solutions on offer, the best roads to life (almost) everlasting currently available.

Glass and the Time Machine

In France in the late-eighteenth century, Pierre Giraud, an architect, had an idea that, in 1801, he explained in a book entitled *Les Tombeaux, ou essai sur les sepultures*. He wished to save the bodies of the dead from dissolution. His idea was based on the discovery that, under the right circumstances, parts of decomposing bodies could turn into glass. This was a natural process, but this was the age of industry. Giraud wished to build a cemetery shaped like a pyramid with a crematorium in the base. The crematorium would reduce bodies to vitrifiable ashes. An entirely new substance would be created – a glass made from human remains. This glass would be used to construct the giant columns of the cemetery's portico and to form memorial portrait medallions and commemorative tablets. The memory of the person would be preserved in the substance of the person.

'How many children would spontaneously, from their earliest youth,' asked Giraud, 'be turned away from the path of crime and dissipation at the mere sight of portraits of their virtuous ancestors?'

This strange idea contains but does not resolve two distinct traditions of thought about death and immortality. The old tradition is that of the morally uplifting memorial designed to inspire future generations. The new tradition is scientific. Giraud wanted to literalise his memorials. They would not just be *about* the person, they would *be* the person. A real presence is offered to future generations instead of the virtual presence of the stone memorial. The idea is unresolved because it is not clear why such an attenuated version of a real presence should strengthen the moral impact of the memorials any more than ordinary stone or marble.

Also in the late-eighteenth century, this time in America, Benjamin Franklin, founding father and polymath, dreamed of the possibility of being preserved at death and brought back to life in the future, '. . . for having a very ardent desire to see and observe the state of America a hundred years hence, I should prefer an ordinary death, being immersed with a few friends in a cask of Madeira until that time, then to be recalled to life by the solar warmth of my dear country. But . . . in all probability, we live in a century too little advanced, and too near the infancy of science, to see such an art brought in our time to perfection.'

(This bodily preservation idea seems to have been in the air at the time. After the Battle of Trafalgar in 1805, the body of Admiral Lord Nelson was returned to Britain preserved in a barrel of brandy. Sailors drank from this barrel in the belief that it would give them some of their commander's courage. And, somewhat later, in 1832, the body of the philosopher

Jeremy Bentham was preserved and kept in a wooden cabinet at University College, London. The whole assembly was known as an Auto-Icon, a superbly clumsy term that could equally well have been applied to Giraud's medallions.)

Both Giraud and Franklin start from the idea that the human body should be preserved. But, from that point, they diverge radically. For Giraud the aim of the project is to inspire future generations. The literalising of the memorial is a tool to this end, not the end in itself. For Franklin, preservation is the whole point. His goal is to see the future and he imagines this being achieved by the resurrection of his body through technology.

Franklin's preservation is a time machine. The period between death and resurrection may be hundreds of years but, to the person involved, the two events will be contiguous. Having been unaware of the intervening darkness, he will feel he has been transported instantly from one time to another. To put this another way: subjective time is a reciprocal of the rate of metabolism; the slower the latter, the faster the former. To the sleeper in suspended animation, centuries pass in the blinking of an eye.

The Big Freeze

Strictly speaking, one Evan Cooper should be called the father of cryonics. In 1962 he published a book called *Immortality, Physically, Scientifically, Now* and, in 1963, he started the Life Extension Foundation in Washington DC. But Cooper was something of an oddity and plainly subject to frustration.

'Are we shouting in the abyss?' he raged in 1964. 'How could 100 million people go to their deaths without one at least, trying for a life in the future via freezing?'

The secretive Cooper became disillusioned with the whole movement and subsequently destroyed all his papers. As a result, the founding father of cryonics – the technology of freezing dead people in order to bring them back to life later – is always seen as Robert Ettinger.

In 1964 Ettinger published *The Prospect of Immortality*. A mathematician and physicist, Ettinger had from childhood been obsessed with the idea of the technological conquest of death. This was to become a highly topical concern. By the time Ettinger was writing, it had become clear that the traditional definition of death – the irreversible cessation of heart and lung function – was inadequate in the context of modern medical technology. Heart and lungs could be kept going artificially. Death began to be seriously reconsidered in 1968 with the report of the Harvard Medical School Ad Hoc Committee and, in 1981, by a US presidential report entitled 'Defining Death'. As a result of this rethinking, the Uniform Determination of Death Act was passed. This established whole brain death – the irreversible cessation of brain functions – as a definition of death, though it did also include the cardiopulmonary definition. Brain death became the more or less universal standard, but the inclusion of the traditional definition left open an area of ambiguity which has led to many celebrated conflicts about individual cases. The legal and philosophical issues raised are, of course, important but, even more important, is the imaginative impact of the *possibility* of such redefinitions. Death had been relativised.

Ettinger saw the implications of this relativisation of death by technology. Somebody once pronounced dead because their heart had stopped could, in a suitably equipped modern hospital, be brought back to life. This suggested that death was culturally defined. Plainly, there was a form of death that all could agree on – say, the total destruction of the body by fire. Lesser degrees of damage, however, could be defined as death in one place and not in others. As technology progressed, ever greater degrees of damage could be sustained without the body being classified as dead. Thus death was not only relative in space – where you were at the moment of crisis – but in time – when you were. Today your lung cancer might be fatal; tomorrow it might not be. To expand this idea to its limit, it might be reasonable to say that if anything survived of the body, then it could not be classified as dead. For example, we know that most cells in our body contain our entire genome in their nucleus. We now know also that adult mammalian cloning is possible. A single cell, therefore, could be used to create a clone of a person. This would be an unsatisfactory form of resurrection because the clone would have none of the constituents of the original's personality – notably its memory. But it does raise the question of what level of damage may be fixable in the future. Death, in short, must now be redefined as simply the point at which current medical technologies are obliged to confess impotence.

Once the future is taken into account and we assume that scientific and technological progress will be limitless, then Benjamin Franklin's time machine becomes a viable proposition. Why shouldn't we project ourselves into the future by any means of preservation we have at our disposal in the hope that whatever is killing or has killed us now will be fixable? This fixing would, of course, include correcting any damage inflicted by the preservation process. A theoretical outline of scientific immortality had been discovered.

Ettinger's book is about the discovery of a preservation process – freezing – and is inspired by an absolute faith in the future as a world of infinite technological competence. Both these themes have some historical resonance. In 1626 Francis Bacon, the great statesman and thinker, died, it is said because he contracted pneumonia after gathering snow to stuff into a chicken. He was convinced, correctly but prematurely, that freezing would preserve meat. The seductive possibilities of the future, meanwhile, not only referred back to Franklin but also to the idea of material progress as a result of the seventeenth-century creation of experimental science. Ettinger simply put two and two together and made four. We should freeze ourselves now to benefit from what would inevitably be a more technologically adept future.

There is, incidentally, plenty of evidence that freezing might, at least in the short term, work. People falling into very cold water have been revived long after, at normal temperatures, they would have suffered terminal brain damage. Experiments at the Safar Center for Resuscitation in Pittsburgh have brought dogs back to life after all heart and brain activity had ceased and they had been cooled to 7 degrees C. It is a technique that could be used with severe battlefield injuries or any major trauma that has caused cardiac arrest. It is, indeed, already used for preserving organs for transplant.

Ettinger's *The Prospect of Immortality* was to become the foundational text of the cryonics movement, which offers to super-cool your body after death and to preserve it until the appropriate technology – both of resurrection and repair but, ideally, also of rejuvenation – becomes available. The book is a remarkable document, whimsical and often wryly prescient, but also insanely utopian. Ettinger sees clearly enough the legal oddity of these frozen entities: 'Heretofore', he observes at one point, 'a corpse has had in itself neither rights nor obligations; now it will have both. His rights will include protection of his body and of his property, governmental supervision of the freezer and of his trust funds. His obligations will include the duty to pay taxes out of his funds and property and to submit his estate to regulation.'

He also raises the curious possibility that failure to freeze somebody may one day be considered a crime. Politically, 'the frozen will constitute an enormous body of influence which must be duly recognized and represented'. Ettinger also discusses intelligently the question of the survival of the self through the preservation process. Indeed, he discusses it intelligently enough to cast doubt on the purpose of the whole enterprise in that we cannot be sure how much of us would survive.

But the blind utopianism overrules all doubts. Blithely, for example, he deals with the population problems that would occur when large-scale resuscitations began:

> ... if we consider the whole world, with a base population of, say, four billion, then the frozen population would increase by four billion every thirty years. If it takes 300 years for civilization to reach the immortality level, there would then be some forty billion people to revive and relocate – if we assume, for simplicity, that it all happens at once ... There is ample room on our planet for forty billion people.

The scientific developments of the fifties and early sixties are used as evidence that we are moving with ever-increasing rapidity into this future. This includes many developments that we now know to have gone nowhere or which have simply been found to be errors. Ettinger, for example, mentions Carrel's strain of chick embryo cells as evidence of our incipient immortality. As I mentioned earlier, this work was thoroughly discredited by Leonard Hayflick.

The final point to make about Ettinger is his complete unconcern with the sort of qualms people feel in contemplating this radically re-engineered future, the sort of qualms they felt – and were intended to feel – about Aldous Huxley's *Brave New World*. He assumes, of course, that the human intellect will have been an aspect of the re-engineering process:

I am convinced that in a few hundred years the words of
Shakespeare, for example, will interest us no more than the
grunting of swine in a wallow . . . Not only will his work
be far too weak in intellect, and written in too vague and
puny a language, but the problems which concerned him
will be, in the main, no more than historical curiosities.
Neither greed, nor lust, nor ambition will in that society
have any recognizable similarity to the qualities we know.

The importance of Ettinger to the contemporary immortalist
movement is comparable to that of Hayflick, Kirkwood, West
or de Grey, but it is different in kind. Though a scientist himself, Ettinger's contribution was not primarily scientific.
Certainly, he inspired the technology of cryonics, but his main
inspiration was conceptual. First, he introduced the idea of
the relativity of death in time and, secondly, he imagined a
world in which death had been conquered and the frozen
resurrected. He imagined this very persuasively. In a crucial
passage, he resurrected the old idea of death as merely a
period of sleep and thereby offered the dying a wondrous
spectacle of hope:

The tired old man, then, will close his eyes, and he can
think of his impending temporary death as another period
under anaesthesia in the hospital. Centuries may pass, but
to him there will be only a moment of sleep without
dreams.

After awakening, he may already be again young and
virile, having been rejuvenated while unconscious; or he
may be gradually renovated through treatment after awakening. In any case, he will have the physique of a Charles
Atlas if he wants it, and his weary and faded wife, if she
chooses, may rival Miss Universe. . . . they will be gradually
improved in mentality and personality. They will not find

themselves idiot strangers in a lonely and baffling world,
but will be made fully educable and integrated.

The excitement of this idea – a technological induction into a
future paradise – has gripped people ever since. Novelists
and technophiles periodically evoke that same moment of
reawakening.

These awakenings have become consolation parables of
the immortalist movement. Ettinger is not just the descendant
of Francis Bacon, but also of the many women writers of the
consolation literature that was so popular in America in the
nineteenth century. Books like Lydia Howard Sigourney's
Margaret and Henrietta, Two Lovely Sisters and Elizabeth
Stuart Phelps's *Between the Gates* and *The Gates Ajar*
assured readers that death was not the end on the basis of
religious faith. Ettinger does so on the basis of scientific faith.
All offer an idealised immortality of transfigured selves and
reunification with loved ones.

The Prospect of Immortality was not, however, to be as
persuasive as Ettinger had hoped. Since its publication, few
people have elected to be frozen and the cryonics business has
lurched from crisis to crisis. Nevertheless, its imaginative
effects have been enormous. Ettinger's thought experiments,
apart from inspiring the immortalist movement, also formed
the basis of science fiction novels like Joe Haldeman's *The
Long Habit of Living* and James L. Halperin's *The First
Immortal*.

What is it that holds us back from embracing the one clear,
rational chance we have of surviving our deaths? Or is it, perhaps, something more exact. Robin Hanson, an economist
who is himself signed up for cryonic suspension, was puzzled
why more people did not also sign up. The reason, he specu-
lates, may be something to do with our primary impulse as a
species to collect 'social allies'. This is done through activities

akin to mutual grooming. We give people, for example, boxes of chocolates not because they might be hungry but to demonstrate our own generosity. Cryonics, however, is utterly devoid of – indeed, counter to – any such process of shoring up alliances.

Hanson writes: 'At present cryonics is something individuals buy for themselves, which if it works, will transport them to an alien social world . . . That alien world seems unattractive and downright scary to most current allies, and spending all that money on going there reduces one's ability to aid current allies. Buying cryonics can then naturally be interpreted as symbolizing one's betrayal and abandonment.'

Even in a highly individualised society, therefore, there is something just too selfish about projecting oneself into an alien future. It means you are prepared to live without the love – alliances in Hanson's terms – of those around you. But not being able to live without it is precisely the sort of term involved in any love contract. And that means an agreement to die together.

None of this held Ettinger back. His not really dead body is now cryo-preserved in liquid nitrogen in Scottsdale, Arizona, as are the bodies of his first wife, Elaine, and his second, Junod.

You Get What You Pay For

Alcor is not in Phoenix but in the suburb of Scottsdale so it cannot quite claim a local affinity with the mythical bird that rises from its own ashes. And, indeed, the bird is no longer the symbol of the company, it has been replaced by a more culturally neutral, futuristic logo. Alcor is the world's leading company in cryonics, but it would be a grave disappointment to Robert Ettinger. When I visited in 2005, there were only sixty-seven individuals – either whole bodies or just heads – in their big, stainless steel Dewars and, though membership had started to rise rapidly – there had been a hundred new applications in the last quarter – there were still only 720 people worldwide signed up for the company's cold time machine. When the Cryonics Institute in Michigan is taken into account, the total number of people signed up for deep freezing is not much more than a thousand. By now, Ettinger would have expected millions or even billions.

Alcor goes to enormous lengths to demonstrate that it is an open and honest company. Cryonics, since Ettinger's book, has had a bumpy ride. The worst incident was in 1979 when nine bodies stored in a cemetery in California thawed out because of lack of funds. Alcor itself has suffered legal problems. The baseball star Ted Williams was frozen there in 2002 but this led to a family dispute over whether it was what he really wanted. And both Alcor and the Cryonics Institute have had legal disputes with their state governments over how their businesses should be classified. Both have survived, though the Cryonics Institute has been forced to reclassify itself as a cemetery. The scars left by these disputes have encouraged Alcor to be almost extravagantly open about its practices.

It is a very small company with few employees. The building is an unremarkable block on a busy road. Alcor has considered purchasing a disused missile silo for the storage of its patients. One reason they haven't done this so far is that they didn't want to be seen as a fringe cult in the desert 'like the Branch Davidians'. If they did ever take in a controversial figure – a famous politican, for example – they would, they admit, have to reconsider the security provisions at their present location.

Inside, the offices are comfortable but nondescript and decorated with pictures of their 'patients' who have not chosen anonymity. Under the pictures are the dates of their 'first life cycle'. Beyond the offices are rooms with equipment for the treatment of whole bodies or just heads. A whole body 'suspension' costs $150,000 and a 'neural' – i.e. just the head – costs $80,000. This makes Alcor more expensive than the Cryonics Institute but, as the then chief executive Joe Waynick explains, 'They're the Volkswagen, we're the Cadillac. You get what you pay for.'

Alcor customers generally pay this through life insurance policies. As I saw on Rudi Hoffman's T-shirt at Atlanta – 'May I bid on your cryonics life insurance?' – this may be a niche business but it's a serious one. But since, as far as the cryonicists are concerned, their patients are not actually dead, might not these insurance policies be considered fraudulent? In fact, I was told, only one insurance company has raised this matter, the rest being content to accept the definition of death currently agreed by the medical profession.

Also behind the offices is the room in which the big, stainless steel Dewars are kept. There are a couple of small ones for pets, but the big ones house a combination of heads and bodies, the latter stored upside down. This is in case there is a loss of the liquid nitrogen coolant. This boils off the top of the Dewars at the rate of about 18 litres per day. If it were not topped up, the level would gradually drop. Storing the bodies upside down means that the head would be the last part to thaw. The whole system is very low maintenance as the Dewars require no power, they simply require regular top-ups. Security, however, needs to be tight. Random vandalism is always possible as is a religious or ideologically inspired attack.

'We encounter a lot of hostility from religious communities,' says my guide Tanya Jones, the chief operating officer, 'a lot of scepticism, a lot of disbelief, it's a very different mindset . . . I've met religious people who think that cryonics is a good thing, I'm very open minded when it comes to stuff like that.'

In fact Waynick, being a Seventh Day Adventist, had worked out the conflicts between Alcor's intentions and those of his religion in conversation with his pastor. His reasoning is a very clear indication of the way in which Americans can so readily combine religious and technological values.

'. . . I had many lively debates with my Pastor. It finally came down to us sitting down . . . and doing some Bible studies on life and death and what it meant in the Scriptures. And we both came to the resolution that there is no Biblical reason why someone cannot participate in a cryonics experiment any more than someone would not want to participate in a heart transplant or why someone would not want to take experimental drugs to try and alleviate the symptoms of an incurable disease? . . .

'I think anything we can do to extend human life is ethical, is imperative . . . Christ was all about healing . . . He taught us we should heal the sick, raise the dead if we could . . . Essentially we are resuscitating people from a very long period of suspended animation and I think that's as close to raising the dead as human beings will ever get. When you go beyond permanent cellular damage, you really are in the purview of God.'

Nevertheless, most Alcor employees and members are, in Jones's words, 'scientifically-minded atheists' who see cryonics as their one chance of survival beyond what we currently call death. It is a chance seized by many in the immortalist business – Aubrey de Grey, for example, is signed up for a neural – and the spreading of the news about possible life-extension technologies available in the near future has led Alcor to believe that they are entering a phase of real growth.

A new 'patient care bay' is being built that would increase their capacity to anything from 300 to 800 patients. On top of the cost of suspension, customers pay $400 a year membership fees. There's another $120 a year in Comprehensive Member Standby – coverage for rescue and transport of members' bodies. Allowing for such revenues and given that each living member is a company asset that will be turned into revenue on death, it is clear that Alcor is a somewhat larger company than these modest premises would suggest. Even so, it needs to grow to give itself a sufficiently high profile to move on to the next stage. Waynick reckons there would be a tipping point at a membership level of 1200, after which Alcor would move to an entirely new rate of growth – perhaps 15 per cent as opposed to their historic level of 8 per cent. The goal is not profit, he insists, but saving lives.

The logistics of the operation are complex. The sooner bodies are cooled and transported to Scottsdale the better. But, obviously, patients can only plan to a limited extent. If they have plenty of prior warning, they can be admitted to a nearby hospital. But death is not always so obliging. For example, Jones says, 'Several of our members were murdered under various circumstances . . . One was a young girl in Spain, twenty-one years old, another was a lawyer shot by one of his clients on the steps of a law library.'

Members wear a bracelet to which doctors and hospitals are supposed to respond by, at the very least, contacting Alcor. If they die in the right place – Florida is good – they will be in reach of one of the trained response teams that will do the right things – cool the body, flush out the blood and so on – immediately after death. They can do nothing before death, however, as this would technically be murder. This is a severe restriction on cryonics as terminal cases may suffer massive brain damage in the process of dying that may limit their chances of a successful resurrection. But only the doctors can decide when enough is enough, not Alcor. This restriction could be removed if cryonics became more widely accepted. 'We wouldn't want to kill anybody,' says Waynick, 'once we are able to demonstrate reversible suspended animation, at that point it would be morally and ethically imperative I think to make the option of elective preservation available. In other words, if you know you have a terminal illness, rather than allow your body to deteriorate to the point where even if you were revivable you would not be right or would require extensive repair work to bring you back to normalcy, going under suspended animation would be a practical and very viable option.'

Cryonics technology itself is changing but remains controversial. For the true believer, of course, the effectiveness of the current technology may be entirely beside the point. It is, after all, the only option available for surviving our doctors' present definition of death and, in any case, now unimaginable, resurrection technologies will be available in the future that will be able to repair whatever damage has been done. The more sceptical will point out that the formation of ice crystals can have a catastrophic effect on cells, ripping open their membranes. A human body will defrost rather in the manner of strawberries, as a soft red goo.

Cryonicists acknowledge that some of the earlier suspensions were technologically crude. Dr James Bedford, frozen in 1967, was the first ever cryonically suspended person. He is in one of the Alcor Dewars and his resurrection, if it ever happens, will be the trickiest of all because he is likely to have suffered considerable damage. It is for this reason that future generations are expected to pursue a last-in first-out policy with cryonics patients – the latest suspensions will be the least damaged.

The best way to overcome damage from ice crystals is to ensure that they never form. This can be done by replacing as much of the body's water as possible with a fluid that does not form crystals but rather turns into a clean, glassy substance at the critical 'glass transition temperature'. This process – known as vitrification – could, when I visited, already be achieved with the brain and Alcor were expecting to soon be able to vitrify the entire body. Pierre Giraud has been vindicated; the way to the future is via glass.

The vitrification technology comes from the California company 21st Century Medicine. I met Greg Fahy from that company at a conference in Cambridge. I brought up the subject of Alcor, but he seemed slightly embarrassed – 'We sent them a few slides.' In fact, the company's main work is in developing vitrification in order to preserve individual organs. The idea here is that stem-cell research may soon mean that we can grow ourselves spare organs. These may be created at birth and then preserved until we needed them. Since they would be, in effect, our own organs, there would be no rejection problem. In that context, the preservation process becomes crucial. Cryonics has effectively piggy-backed on this technology.

So, on the face of it, both through current technology and through new expectations of future technologies, cryonics seems to be increasingly well-placed. Furthermore, as an industry it seems to have survived suspicions about its motives, its practices and accusations that it is a cultish or even blasphemous procedure. The emphasis at Alcor was on persuading me of the sanity and normality of the whole oper-ation and of its customers. They are not, I was assured, undignified cowards or obsessive hypochondriacs, but, rather, optimistic, positive people who loved life too much to turn down an opportunity of prolonging it. Furthermore, if people still want to die after they have been woken up, at least they will have the choice to do so on their own terms.

'My mother does not want to sign up for cryonics', says Tanya Jones, 'because she doesn't want to do this all over again, she's tired – she's fifty-nine – I feel bad for her, she's had a rough life but I don't think that's any reason to give up now. But there are people who will take their own lives, I just think it will be with a heck of a lot more dignity than they are afforded today.'

Cryonics represents the most literal bid for immortality available today. It is surprising it has not been more successful in attracting customers. Perhaps it will now do so. But, meanwhile, there a number of other options you can pursue to keep you going.

Thin People

You see a lot of thin people at immortality and life-extension conferences – not thin in the sense of slim or not fat, but thin in the sense of alarmingly etiolated. Some appear to be unable to buy clothes that fit them, their slender necks emerge from excessively large collars and their trousers are only just held up by thick belts. One thin man I saw escape from the confines of a Cambridge conference in order, apparently, to hide behind a wall. On following him, I saw that he was conducting some form of meditation that involved a strange, one-legged posture. This went on for some time, so I abandoned my stake-out. Later, I saw him behind me in the conference hall nervously consulting his watch. At the right moment, he took out some pills from a bottle in his pocket and swallowed a handful. Prolonging your life is hard, disciplined and, gastronomically at least, unrewarding work.

Such people sometimes inspire interest and enthusiasm from their colleagues, but, equally often, derision or even contempt. 'Those are the real religious fanatics,' one doctor whispered to me, gesturing at a group of pale wraiths in baggy clothes. These are the disciples of Calorie Restriction (CR) who pursue longevity by placing themselves on a permanent and very strict diet.

This idea has a long history. The Taoists, as I have mentioned, believed that a restricted diet was one essential aspect of the pursuit of immortality. Similarly, Luigo Cornaro, a celebrated pursuer of a longer, healthier life in Italy in the fifteenth century, advocated very careful dieting in his book *Discorsi della Vita Sobria*. Cornaro, like many before and after, believed that we aged and died because of the expenditure of a substance – an 'innate moisture' or 'vital principle' – of which we were given a fixed quantity at birth, enough, in Cornaro's terms, for a hundred years of life. People, he believed, should eat very small quantities and only of food that agreed with them. These quantities would decrease in old age because, he believed, old people required less fuel. A curious and important aspect of Cornaro was his specific justification for the pursuit of longevity:

'Our Maker, having ordained that the life of man should last for many years, is desirous that everyone should attain the extreme limit; since He knows that, after the age of eighty, man is wholly freed from the bitter fruits of sensuality ... Then, of necessity, vices and sins are left behind. Wherefore it is that God wishes we should all live to extreme age.'

Old age is more holy because all passion is spent. There is an austere puritanism at work here. The intake of food, in this context, becomes something we should pursue as an unfortunate necessity rather than a sensuous pleasure. Food, it seems, is a messy invasion of our inner, God-given purity. This was to become an even more literal obession in the mind of the Russian microbiologist Elie Metchnikoff, a Nobel prizewinner in 1908. Metchnikoff believed problems lay with the bacterial swamp of the large intestine. This was an evolutionary hangover that left us subject to constant bacterial invasion. It was this disgusting mess that eventually killed us. Again there is the idea that we have some inner purity that is compromised by our lower, animal natures. This has links with the idea of the soul, of course, but, in this context, it is not so much a freeing of our essence from our bodies as a restoring of the body to its original purity. Irrespective of what science may be involved, these ideas seem to be an expression of a permanent human longing to free ourselves from our earthly ancestry.

But science was to become seriously involved in 1934 when Clive M. McCay's team at Cornell University announced that laboratory rats on a restricted calorie diet lived as much as twice as long as rats fed a normal diet. The diets contained normal amounts of nutrients, it was only the calories that were restricted. As Leonard Hayflick points out, these rats were thus not malnourished, they were undernourished.

It was not immediately clear what this proved. Obviously, lab rats live better lives than rats in the wild. They can eat all that they want. In the wild, they will suffer periodic bouts of famine. Perhaps, therefore, McCay had returned their diets to their more natural condition and that was why they lived longer. They would be unlikely to live longer in the wild, of course, because predation and disease would kill them before they could feel benefit from their diet. Nevertheless, the experiment might simply be one more demonstration of the life-shortening affects of the affluent, high-calorie, low-exercise lifestyle. The rats in captivity were, as they so often are, symbols of modern man.

That would be enough to prove the benefits of a more austere food regime but it would not prove that calorie restriction was desirable in itself. Or it could be desirable if it works by reducing overall metabolic rate and thus the accumulation of toxic products in the body. This would link it to the old idea of, among others, Cornaro that we aged and died more quickly as a result of an excessive rate of living. This metabolic slowdown may be a defence mechanism of organisms. In times of famine, they shut down bodily activity to conserve energy. Life extension would simply be a side-effect.

The Hormesis Hypothesis of CR is more complex. This arises from the discovery that certain types of very low intensity stress can actually protect an organism. 'Moderate stress extends the life span of yeast about 30 per cent,' reports *Scientific American*. It is possible that the stress produced by a restricted calorie diet actually stimulates defensive responses that improve general health and slow ageing. Other studies have suggested that the low calorie intake is not the issue at all, rather it is the preservation of a lean body. This can be achieved by a reduction in insulin uptake, so it is conceivable that all the benefits of CR could be achieved without actually dieting.

Whatever the explanation, calorie restriction has been shown to extend the lives of a number of species. It also seems to improve their health. Monkeys on CR, for example, don't seem to get diabetes, a condition that afflicts half of normally fed monkeys. The indications are strong, therefore, that it would work in humans, though obviously this is hard to prove as any experiment would take decades as well as being ethically dubious. There would be risks involving, for example, brain damage that might not have been apparent in the animals. There can, therefore, be no official medical endorsement of dietary restriction, though, of course, all doctors recommend some control of diet and the avoidance of obesity.

What Robert Ettinger is to cryonics, Roy Walford is to calorie restriction. Having realised this fairly on in my researches, I sought him out on the Internet. Sadly, I soon came across his obituary. Walford died, aged seventy-nine, of respiratory failure, a complication arising from a form of motor neurone disease, in 2004. Walford had been Professor of Pathology at the University of California at Los Angeles and, among other achievements, he spent two years as crew physician in Biosphere 2, the experimental closed community in Arizona. His enthusiasm for calorie restriction proved helpful in the biosphere when it became clear that the crew could not grow as much food as they expected.

On the foundation of the McCay experiments, Walford constructed a whole way of life around the life-extending benefits of calorie restriction. In the introduction to his book *Beyond the 120 Year Diet*, he acknowledges the developments in human biology that may lead to extended lives, but he adds that we cannot possibly know when these might turn into available treatments. And so . . .

> . . . what can we do in the meantime to enhance our chances of still being alive and vital when the more sophisticated techniques arrive? . . . Calorie restriction with optimal nutrition, which I call the 'CRON Diet', will retard your rate of ageing, extend life span (up to perhaps 150 to 160 years, depending on when you start and how thoroughly you hold to it), and markedly decrease susceptibility to most major diseases.

Walford inspired a movement similar to cryonics. Through, for example, the Calorie Restriction Society, you can attend conferences at which almost all the people will be alarmingly thin and you can swap recipes. The dietary regimes both in Walford's book and those suggested by various CR groups look basically the same as those recommended simply for losing weight. The big difference is that slimmers will only expect to be on such diets for a few months, the CR diets are for life.

This is very demanding and also risky if pursued too enthusiastically. Walford mentions a 'fad diet' that emerged in the 1970s called 'The Last Chance Diet'. This involved a liquid

protein intake of 300–400 calories a day. Several people who
were on this for between two to eight months died of heart
failure. They could, at the last, console themselves with a 30
to 50 per cent weight loss. The CR Society warns of a number
of dangers including choking – because of 'CR-induced eat-
quickly psychology' – anaemia, discomfort when sitting on
hard surfaces, loss of libido, slower wound healing and,
unsurprisingly, hunger.

In fact, the base line CR diet involves intake of between
1100 and 1500 calories a day. This compares with the average diet of between 2400 and 3200 calories for men and
1600 to 2200 for women. What is actually eaten must be as
rich in nutrients as possible and any rapid weight loss should
be slowed by an increase in calories. The trick is moderation
for, as the CR Society website warns, 'Taken to extremes or
practiced without due caution, unbalanced CR practice may
result in a person losing his/her life in order to save it.'

Benjamin Colby, Emeritus Professor in Anthropology at
the University of California, was when I met him a very thin
and healthy looking seventy-three-year-old. Having read
Walford, he consumes about 1500 calories, runs along the
beach and works out two or three times a day. He admits the
science of CR is uncertain. It is not known, for example,
when is the optimum time to start. Very young people might
have their growth damaged, but it is not clear whether starting CR in old age gives any benefit at all.

'Evidence suggests', he says, 'that even late starters may
have some advantage. But my main concern is not so much
extension of life as quality. If we are able to be productive up
until the end, then it's worth it.'

Colby is very well; he was once told he had the vascular
system of a teenager. He is, however, somewhat concerned
about osteoporosis – loss of bone mass leading to fragility –
resulting from his diet. This may well be a risk and it did

occur in CR monkeys. However, Colby thinks, along with other CR enthusiasts, that, though there may be loss of bone mass, this is compensated for by greater bone strength. He is an exemplary CR figure, not fanatical and not prone to hiding behind walls.

CR is gaining credibility. In 2006, a study was reported in the *Journal of the American College of Cardiology* which claimed to be the first to link low calorie diets with delayed ageing in humans. Scientists at Washington University School of Medicine had used ultrasound to study the hearts of twenty-five people who had been maintaining a CR diet of between 1400 and 2000 calories a day for a minimum of six years. Their condition was measured against twenty-five people who had been on a standard 'Western' diet of between 2000 and 3000 calories a day. The CR subjects had more elastic hearts and fewer signs of incipient disease than the control group. The study is far from conclusive, but it does provide circumstantial evidence that what has been found to be true of animals might also be true of humans – eating less makes you live longer.

Cryonics and CR have much in common. They both have a symbolically potent founder figure – Ettinger and Walford – and they are both concerned with deferring the diagnosis of death until new technologies come along. Cryonics is somewhat less scientifically respectable as CR is supported by plenty of non-human experimental evidence and there is, as yet, no evidence that cryonics can work. On the other hand, cryonics makes a much more substantial promise. Whereas CR simply promises that, if you keep at this punishing regime, you might survive long enough to benefit from new technologies, cryonics says that, if it works, it offers the total defeat of death, for the moment at least.

They have one further and much more important thing in common. They require commitment – a decision to believe and to devote time and effort to acting on that belief – and sacrifice – financial in the case of cryonics and sensuous in the case of CR. To shore up this sacrificial aspect, both these longevity institutions are at pains to insist on the ethical rightness of what they are doing and the essential healthiness and optimism of their participants. These people are not cowards, afraid of death, they are heroes, in love with life.

The Me Generation

Cryonics and CR were the forerunners of what was to become, in the late sixties and seventies, a consumerist death-avoidance programme. This was inspired by discoveries like the dangers of smoking, high cholesterol, a sedentary lifestyle and an inadequate diet. Such scientific insights had been around for some time but the message did not sink in until the consumers were ready to hear it. They were made ready by the glorification of the self, the ideology behind the libertarian and liberationist movements of the late sixties and, ultimately, the immortalist movement.

The Cold War was a real war. It was fought through surrogates in Vietnam and Korea, but it also involved keeping civilian populations at home on a war footing. I remember sombre discussions and pamphlets about what would happen and what we must do in the event of a nuclear strike. I was aware of Soviet bombers probing our defences over the North Sea and, both on television and in my dreams, I saw ICBMs rising irrevocably out of their silos in the American West. In my bedroom, I kept a *Scientific American* picture of all the missiles in the US arsenal.

There was an external enemy, ready and willing to kill us all at a moment's notice – to be exact, in the case of Britain, four minutes' notice. This had a stifling effect. It imposed a feeling that, as during the war of 1939–45, we must conform and obey in the name of national survival. People rebelled – the existentialists, angry young men and beats in the fifties, the teens with their anti-parent music in the fifties and sixties, the civil rights movements of the sixties – but these were disparate and specialised rebellions. The rejection of Cold War conformity and mutuality finally coalesced into an ideology of the self in the late sixties, most obviously in the 'Summer of Love' in 1967.

To insist on the primacy of the self is an anti-war gesture. War, after all, can only occur if the self can be sacrificed, if it sees itself as an aspect or instrument of something greater. What failed in the late sixties was the concept of 'something greater'. This may, in the first two decades of the Cold War, have been seen as the nation, freedom or civilisation, but, at the beginning of the third decade, it came to be interpreted as a paranoid construct. It consisted of the military-industrial complex, of secretive organisations like the CIA, of capitalism in general and of corporate life in particular. With the intractable carnage of Vietnam, the 'something greater' that justified war stopped being a benign nexus and became the malign one known as 'The System'.

The self opposed itself to The System through now very familiar mechanisms of clothes, protests, demonstrations, sit-ins, music, drugs and a whole syllabus of alternative cultural references. Emerging from this was the self-centred project of the 'lifestyle'. Having a lifestyle implied a choice, it meant that you did not accept the way of life imposed or required by The System. It meant that the activities you pursued and the objects by which you were surrounded were now to be aspects, not of Cold War, survivalist mutuality, but of the project of your own self-actualisation.

Lifestyle conscripted to its cause the medical science that had begun to show us what was wrong with our old, System-led existence. Conventionally clad, nicotine-dosed, fat-laden, zero-exercised, high-stressed lives were creations of The System. Now we knew that this war-based system was killing its own people by making them consume and behave in fatal ways. Rejecting such patterns became as much of a protest against The System as a civil-rights or anti-war march or smoking dope. Choosing to live longer had become part of the alternative culture.

All of which explains very precisely the career of Jane Fonda. Fonda used her fame as a Hollywood star to publicise her opposition to the Vietnam War, a process that came to a climax with her visit to Hanoi in 1972. There she posed next to anti-aircraft guns and said she wished she had American planes in her sights. She became Hanoi Jane, the heroine ready to pitch her own self and its conscience against The System and its war machine.

Her second attack on The System was less dramatic but more profitable. In 1979 she started the Jane Fonda Workout Studio in Los Angeles. Her various exercise regimes were then put on video. From *Workout* (1982) through *Prime Time Workout* (1985), *Lower Impact Aerobic Workout* (1986), *Toning and Shaping* (1987), *Lower Body Solution* (1991) right up to *Abs, Buns and Thighs* (1995), Fonda bounded about in her leotards, showing the people of the world how to reject the bad old ways of The System and embrace The Lifestyle.

There is nothing new about cultish exercise regimes – both modernist architects and fascist dictators had embraced them in the thirties as necessary aspects of Utopia – but Fonda's was the version for the 'Me' generation. It was all about taking control of the body and, therefore, the self and about fighting off the fatal depredations of modern life. Her fame, combined with the home video machine, institutionalised exercise for the post-System generation. Fonda inspired people with the idea that our lives could be controlled by our own wills, controlled and, more to the point, extended.

Erotic Self-Image Plays a Major Role in Neuroendocrine Production

In 1982, Durk Pearson and Sandy Shaw produced an astonishing 858-page book entitled *Life Extension: A Practical Scientific Approach*. The sub-sub-heading on the front cover was 'Adding Years to Your Life and Life to Your Years'. The book takes the health cult of the Me generation to its logical conclusion. What is on offer here are not just better years but more of them. Pearson and Shaw introduced life extension to a mass audience. They continue to do so through *Life Enhancement* magazine and nutritional supplements.

The continuity from the Fonda to the Pearson/Shaw approach is evident in the book's illustrations. The authors are shown in various unclad or partly clad poses. A naked Durk, his genitals concealed by surfboard, and a leotard-wearing Sandy, face each other on two pages. The caption summarises the way the sacrificial aspects of the regime they recommend – diet, exercise, a constant intake of supplements – is balanced by the sensual good life enjoyed by devoted followers. They write: 'Erotic self-image plays a major role in neuroendocrine function. (Youthful erotic stimulation has been shown to alter the neuroendocrine systems of old male and female rats and rhesus monkeys towards more youthful function.) Not only is staying young good for your sex life, a good sex life can help you stay young.'

There are two further photographs of Durk, naked but for a posing pouch, in muscle man poses. The caption here reads: 'I'd rather eat growth hormone releasing nutrients than exercise. My 13 per cent body fat is close to the 12.4 per cent average for male athletes who are world class swimmers. Can life extenders do it longer in the sun? Yes, you can be in the sun longer without burning when you use singlet oxygen quenchers and free radical scavenging antioxidants. Anyone for a romp in the desert?'

This is the familiar win-win rhetoric – you live longer AND it's more fun – that is now so familiar from chat shows, advertisements, self-help books and celebrity autobiographies. It is a self-sustaining idea. In the 1930s, for example, a muscled body like Sandy Pearson's would not have been seen as attractive in a woman. But, if a worked, gym-fit look is made fashionable, then pursuing that look does more than make you healthy, it makes you socially acceptable. You can't lose.

The book itself is a bewildering collection of recommendations, cautions and warnings based on the prevailing medical wisdom and speculation of the time. Much of it was derived from the free radical theory of ageing proposed by Deham Harman in the late fifties. This suggested that ageing was caused by the accumulation of damage caused by unstable compounds produced by oxygen reactions, notably with fats. But the crucial point about the book's approach is the way it attempted to subvert the medical expertise embodied in the medical establishment. Although Pearson and Shaw repeatedly recommend formal consultations with one's doctor, they also recommend developing a massive programme of self-prescription and they repeatedly attack the Federal Drug Administration for its conservatism about the beneficial effects of many drugs. Later they were to be involved in legal action with the FDA on this issue.

The wider significance of the book is its relentless exposition of the idea that enough is now known for us to take charge of our own longevity. Pearson and Shaw repeatedly address themselves to people of 'above average intelligence' and they make it clear that the regime they are advocating has to be approached with a degree of devotion beyond the capacities and understanding of most people.

They also make it clear that the uninformed and the idle will be denied life-extension technology not just by their own shortcomings but also by medical and scientific institutions:

The Food and Drug Administration (FDA) does not approve drugs specifically for life extension, and the approval of a new drug for conventional anti-disease purposes takes eight to twelve years, on the average. The scientific information upon which the drugs have been based will generally be known many years before any practical applications may be offered in the American marketplace.

In other words, there is an institutional conspiracy to keep the information from the people. After Vietnam and Watergate and with Iran-Contra soon to burst open, this was an idea for which the people were well-prepared. Mistrust of even democratic governments was becoming one of the great political and cultural forces of the post-war world.

This conviction – that we could extend our lives if only governments would let us – continues to inspire people today. It usually manifests itself in claims from enthusiasts for nutritional supplements that official inertia or incompetence is refusing to acknowledge the benefits of. That's certainly the battle Pearson and Shaw continued to fight.

The problem the authorities have, of course, is that they cannot say definitively that any supplement or regime does *not* extend your life. They can only say, as they do, that the evidence is non-existent, inadequate or inconclusive. This problem is compounded by the fact that, much as the medical establishment may wish to distance itself from promises of life extension, that is, in fact, the very game it is in. All medicine tries to stop you dying, that is its primary function. Science has created the expectation, but now finds itself having to regulate its popular expression.

Obviously, it must fail in this task because the expectation is so huge and what science now appears to be offering is relatively minor in comparison. People have only a limited amount of time in which to take evasive action against death. Many of the promises of medical science, however, seem to be receding into an ever more remote future – notably the cure for cancer which has been confidently promised for more than fifty years. This is because the great life-extending break-throughs of the twentieth century cannot easily be repeated and the pace of improvement in life expectancy cannot necessarily be maintained. This creates the now familiar anxiety that people alive today will miss out. It is hardly surprising, therefore, that people go to great lengths and great expense to defy official medical wisdom and to seek out alternatives. After all, the elixir of life may already be wending its tortuous way through government bureaucracy and, as it does so, people are dying for lack of it.

The Self-Dosers

This puts babyboomer doctors and scientists with immortalist tendencies in a tricky position. They may be firmly convinced that some procedures will indeed extend life, but officialdom may prevent them from prescribing them for their patients. It does not, however, prevent them from prescribing for themselves.

At Cambridge, one scientist told me that, though he did not have a cholesterol problem, he took high doses of statins, cholesterol-lowering drugs. Also, though his blood pressure was not high, he took drugs to lower it even further. He was maintaining his resting systolic pressure at 100. A healthy adult resting systolic pressure is reckoned to be about 120. A doctor by my side was horrified. He pointed out that we need a certain level of cholesterol and very low blood pressure could lead to strokes. Certainly, at 100 or below it could make your life very unpleasant with bouts of fainting and dizziness. The scientist was unmoved. The evidence suggested that life would be extended by much lower cholesterol and the blood pressure. He was aware, of course, that it would be entirely unethical – and, indeed, illegal – to prescribe such treatments for the population at large.

In fact, almost everybody in the immortality business seems to engage in some form of self-dosing. For example, at Cambridge Greg Fahy of 21st Century Medicine in California had given me an explanation of his technology of preserving organs through vitrification – the process now used by Alcor –and I asked him what he did to stay alive. There was the usual diet and exercise formula but then he pulled a bag full of pills out of his trouser pocket. There were multi-vitamins, a 'life-extension mix', anti-inflammatories and so on. It was a fairly normal cocktail in this business.

Self-dosing draws attention to an ethical curiosity. On the whole, medicines do not become available until their safety is more or less guaranteed. When death is imminent, of course, some relaxation occurs and potent drugs are administered that might damage a healthy person. But, from another perspective, death is imminent for all of us all of the time. Our increasing knowledge of killers like heart disease and cancer has shown that they often begin years before they show any symptoms and certainly long before death. In particular, certain inflammatory conditions that would once have been regarded as trivial are now known to be the seeds of our destruction. Once they pass a certain age, all our bodies are busily engaged in the process of dying. Perhaps we are all so close to death that we can demand a degree of ethical relaxation. Of course, we can all self-dose with supplements and vitamins. But only doctors have access to those compounds known to be the most effective. How many of them exploit that privilege is unclear.

'All of them,' I was told at one point.

The Supreme Boomer

Having been in contact with his office a couple of times, I get a lot of Ray Kurzweil material. Two enormously fat books – *Fantastic Voyage* and *The Singularity is Near* – have arrived since I started writing this one. There are periodic e-mails. For a while, as a result of a bug in his computer, I started receiving e-mails he had sent to other people. This gave me a glimpse into the life of a busy, energetic and distinctly in-demand man.

Kurzweil is, in fact, an emblematic figure, the supreme embodiment of a peculiarly American belief in the future. He is a multiply-honoured author and inventor of, among other things, a system for enabling computers to read, the Kurzweil 250 electric piano which sounds like a concert grand, a computer speech recognition system, a financial system aimed at producing an artificially intelligent stock analyst and so on. He is perhaps the leading prophet of the imminent Singularity when technological acceleration and convergence will take us beyond the human world and, of course, he wants to live forever.

In 1993, he published his second book, *The 10% Solution for a Healthy Life: How to Eliminate Virtually All Risk of Heart Disease and Cancer*. This was based on his successful nutritional programme of self-treatment for type II diabetes. In 2004 with Terry Grossman, he published *Fantastic Voyage: Live Long Enough to Live Forever*.

Kurzweil is also the supreme boomer – he was born on

12th February 1948. In *Fantastic Voyage*, he notes the perilous position of his generation, standing, as it does, on the 'critical threshold' of life-extension technology. 'A small minority of older boomers will make it past this impending critical threshold. You can be among them . . . Unfortunately most of our fellow baby boomers remain oblivious to the hidden degenerative processes inside their bodies and will die unnecessarily young.'

The boomers are 'the last generation in which the vast majority will die in the more or less "old fashioned" way, generally from debilitating progressive conditions that severely interfere with the quality of life'. Until the technology comes along, however, the boomers have to be very very careful. They must treat their good health as a constant, proactive project, not something you only notice when you are sick: 'Health is not simply the absence of disease; rather, it refers to the effectiveness of every level of your existence, something you can always improve. The effort you put into this endeavour will be repaid many times and will assist you in whatever life goals you may have.'

The effort is considerable. Kurzweil sees it as a military campaign – 'it's important to have good intelligence on the enemy'. The first step is a genes test followed by constant monitoring of blood levels. His regime of taking supplements – he prefers to call them nutritionals – is punishing, involving 250 pills a day. He also spends one day a week at a complementary medicine clinic. And so on.

The hermetic intensity of such a regime provokes the obvious thought: what is the point of devoting so much energy to staying alive, energy that could be better spent living? The answer is that the regime is a temporary expedient intended to carry Kurzweil, alive and in good health, to the safety of the farther shore where microbiology and nanotechnology will make him medically immortal. A few decades of obsessive body maintenance would then be rewarded with centuries of carefree existence later. As *Fantastic Voyage* concludes: 'There is really no alternative.'

In reviewing this book in *Nature*, Tom Kirkwood observes that, in Britain, the Cancer Act of 1939 is still extant. This act outlaws any advertisement offering 'to treat any person for cancer, or to prescribe any remedy therefore, or to give any advice in connection with the treatment thereof'. The act was plainly to prevent hucksters exploiting the gullible with false hopes. There is no equivalent act against claims for anti-ageing treatments. Kirkwood is certainly not accusing Kurzweil of hucksterism – he says the book does 'a fair job of summarizing the current state of knowledge about factors that can affect the ageing process and about what can sensibly be done to increase your chances of living into old age in good health'. But he is concerned about the hype and with the message that you must do this because it may mean you will live forever. That way leads to obsession, whereas both the Cancer Act and the sane acceptance of the best medical knowledge – on exercise, obesity etc. – should lead to good health and realism about one's prospects.

There is a deep gulf here between the boosters of immortality and the mainstream scientists, between those who believe any gamble on any promising regime, however demanding, is justified and those who see, instead, the dangers of raising false hopes. The problem is that, even in the mainstream, life extension is on the cards and the only alternative to hopes, however false, is the unthinkable extinction of the self.

Fish Oil

For people with normal lives and appetites and limited funds, none of these alternatives, least of all Kurzweil's, may seem

attractive. Freezing, starving, self-dosing or living in a perpetual state of self-administered intensive care all seem to be
very high prices to pay. Speaking as somebody who can't
even remember to take one low-dose aspirin a day – generally
regarded as an uncontentious and risk-free precaution for
men of my age – I cannot begin to imagine leading a life like
Kurzweil's. I am more inclined to the school of medicine
advocated by the wicked Dr Kelso in the TV series *Scrubs*.
For Kelso the good life consists of a 16-ounce steak and a fist-
ful of blood thinners – binge eating combined with binge
medication.

The price of survival by any of these methods seems even
higher when the likelihood of success is taken into account. It
is neither certain that cryonics will work nor that future generations will have any interest in reviving us. Calorie
restriction may still prove to be catastrophic in humans. And
all the various self treatments are subject to opposing scientific opinion. Finally, if life-extension technology is a hundred
years in the future as opposed to thirty, then, no matter what
steps you take, you're not likely to make it to a hundred,
never mind a thousand.

Nevertheless, it would take steel nerves and a locked imagination not to succumb to the pressure of the daily downpour
of health advice and advertising aimed at preserving youth
and avoiding death. But there is so much of it that it is impossible to be sure which makes sense and which doesn't.
Furthermore, our increasing knowledge of the human
genome has made it clear that very few drugs, supplements,
regimes or even resolutions – like giving up smoking – are
universally effective. Tiny variations in our genomes, known
as snips (single nucleotide polymorphisms) are now thought
to lead to massive variations in our responses to any treatment. In the future, it is thought drugs will be tailored
precisely to our own DNA. Equally, we may be able to

establish that some people can eat, drink, smoke and take no exercise to their heart's content because their genome protects them.

For the time being, however, we have the fish oil problem.

As I rose early one morning to work on this chapter, a news story about fish oil popped up on my computer.

'There is no evidence', said the BBC News intro, 'of clear benefits to health from fats which are commonly found in oily fish, researchers say.'

A meta-study had found that omega-3 fatty acids, those found in oily fish like salmon and mackerel, may not be as unconditionally good for us as we had previously thought. People already with heart disease actually seemed to be made worse by fish oil.

'Looking at 3,114 men with stable angina in 2003 it found that those given high amounts of oily fish were at a higher risk of heart attack and recorded an increased number of cardiac deaths.'

Two days earlier, there had been another story about fish oil on the BBC website. 'A diet rich in a fat found in oily fish may protect men with prostate cancer from developing a more aggressive form of the disease, scientists have found.'

These stories are not contradictory – chronic heart disease and prostate cancer are two quite different things and fish oil may make the former worse and the latter better. Furthermore, even after the second story appeared, casting doubt on the benefits to the heart of fish oil, scientists were still insisting that, for people without chronic heart disease, omega-3s were beneficial.

Nevertheless, the lay imagination is likely to be troubled. Carried around in the mind of the normally aware person in the developed world are a number of what are taken to be scientifically sound insights into the structure of the healthy life. These will range all the way from what appear to be near certainties – like the benefits of not smoking, taking exercise, eating a lot of fruit and vegetables, little red meat, lots of whole grains and plenty of oily fish – to the distinctly uncertain and largely faith-based – various dietary supplements, herbal remedies and numerous anti-stress, anti-cancer and generally anti-death procedures.

Fish oils had been up at the near-certainty end of this list for some time, perhaps not as well-established as not smoking but right up there with taking exercise and cutting down on red meat. So deeply embedded are such ideas in the mind of the average layman that he will actually feel better the moment he tastes a forkful of salmon just as he does when he steps on the treadmill. Once the idea took hold that we could control our physical destinies, then we made ourselves open to the daily absorption of certain types of news from the laboratories. In addition, specific aspects of the idea are further reinforced by advertising. For example, we seem, currently, to be in the midst of an advertising blitz on the benefits of whole grains, bran is always being forced through our colons and a vast industry sells us running shoes.

The effect of which is to generate an excess of certainty. So much so that, when I first saw the negative fish oil story, I found myself thinking, 'That can't be true!' But why should I think that? I had not invented the notion that fish oils were good and no blinding revelation had given me faith. Science had told me one thing and now it was telling me something else. The story made me feel like Miles Monroe in the film *Sleeper* (Woody Allen, 1973). Monroe wakes up 200 years in the future and is immediately offered a cigarette. There is, he is told, nothing better for him. It may happen. Science is provisional, its insights always subject to qualification. Even smoking may not be unambiguously bad for you, there has been some suggestion it protects against Parkinson's disease. Too much fish may increase your risk from certain viruses and from mercury poisoning and avoiding caffeine by drinking herbal teas can be damaging either through impurities or excess. You can get as sick from being too thin as from being too fat. Your chances of having a heart attack during exercise soar tenfold and too much exercise increases your risk from free radical damage. Damaso Crespo, a Spanish neurologist, told me it was better to walk a hundred yards than to run as long as you walked and talked with a friend. Exercising the brain is much more important than exercising the body. The brain rots whatever happens to the body and it is well known – or is at the moment – that keeping mentally active staves off some of the rot. But then, of course, mental activity might lead to stress which can cause heart problems.

Does this mean that we know nothing, that nothing can be done, will ever be done?

Be Nice, Be Thin, Have Daughters

Much depends, of course, on our enthusiasm for the project. At one end of the range is Kurzweil, at the other is the fat slob slumped in front of the TV game show. Somewhere in the middle are you, me and Dr Kelso. In the middle, our assessment of the efficacy of the project, the fear of death – or simply prolonged ill-health – and our possibly damaging appetites for life all combine to create our personal contract, the deal we make with what we fear, know and want. Kelso's ideal dinner – steak and blood thinners – is just a comedy version of what we all, the slob excepted, do daily.

On that basis, neither I nor any of the scientists or doctors I have met can be of much help. Some things seem to be known with something close to certainty, but, as the fish oil story demonstrates, that certainty can collapse in an instant. In addition, any of these measures are subject to the peculiarities of your genetic inheritance. Even not smoking may do you no good if you happen to have some particular combination of genes that makes you immune to its effects – or, more accurately, the damage done by smoking would not kill you because other things would do so first. And, finally, there are your own inclinations, whether, unlike me, you can remember to take so much as a low-dose aspirin every day. Thwarting these inclinations with some strict health regime may do you more harm than good.

That said, it is clear that how you live your life will, to some extent, determine when you die. Swedish research in the nineties on identical twins suggested that our genes are far less important than we might think. Identical twins have exactly the same genes and so should, in theory, die at about the same time. But they don't. Indeed, the varying death rates discovered by the Swedes indicated that our genes are only about 20 to 30 per cent responsible for determining the hour of our death. Equally, studies of Seventh Day Adventists in Utah – they don't touch alcohol, caffeine or tobacco – showed they lived on average eight years longer than Americans in general. Diet may also account for the phenomenal longevity of the Japanese living on the islands of Okinawa. The population is 1.3 million and 600 of them have made it past a hundred, the highest density of centenarians in the world. Research has shown that Okinawans exercise a great deal and eat a low-salt, low-fat diet of fruit, vegetables and a staggering amount of soya which is thought to combat cancer. There may, however, be a genetic explanation as they have been found to have variations in the human leukocyte antigen genes that may make them less vulnerable to autoimmune diseases like lupus, rheumatoid arthritis and multiple sclerosis.

The other big site for contemporary hyperborean legends of longevity is Sardinia. In 1999 a team of researchers found

66 people aged a hundred or more in the Nuoro province with a population of 280,000 – three times the Western average. Again it seems to be a case of exercise and diet with the additional ingredient of red wine. Perversely, there also seems to be a generally bleak outlook on life among the Sardinians. This may help to reduce stress and it is, of course, the exact opposite of the sunny disposition generally regarded as a good thing among American immortalists.

The problem is that the fever for life extension means that there are many claims but little evidence. In general, I have concluded that most procedures that are currently claimed to extend your life will not, in fact, do so. This includes those of mainstream medicine as well as those of alternative therapies and the various forms of diet supplementation on offer. This is not a scientific conclusion, it is merely an intuition acquired from listening and reading to all that is said and written in this area. You may live longer than your parents, probably longer than your grandparents and almost certainly longer than your great-grandparents. But this will be due to a continuing, general rise in life expectancy which is, in its most recent phase, not fully understood. If it is a process you can influence, then it will probably be through the methods I list below. But don't count on it.

Even if none of them actually extend your life, that is not a reason not to pursue some of these remedies. Some, though they may not make you live longer, may make you live better. If you have a morning cough and find yourself choking on phlegm, it's probably a good idea to stop smoking even if its effect on you may not be fatal. If you find yourself out of breath after a dozen or so stair treads, then you will feel better and more capable if you exercise. If you're fat, diet because obesity makes everything more difficult and because the sight of a very fat man being given a special extension to his seat belt on a plane is almost unbearably sad. Here, therefore, are a few general procedures that seem to be worth doing.

Exercise appears to work. This is not as obvious as it sounds. Apart from being crushed by a dumb-bell or breaking your neck on a treadmill, there are two important ways in which exercise can kill you. First, your chances of a heart attack while exercising are enormously higher than when not exercising. Secondly, exercise increases the production of free radicals, thus raising your chances of, among other things, cancer. On the other hand, the benefits of exercise are clear – weight loss, better general health and so on. The heart issue is somewhat resolved by the fact that those who exercise have, when not exercising, a lower risk of heart disease than those who don't. In other words, you trade off your higher risk when exercising for the lower risk when not exercising. The trick is not to exercise too much or too violently or the balance of risk moves against you. The same applies to the matter of free radical production. Excessive exercise will tip the risk scales to the point where the risk of free radical damage outweighs the benefits. In short, the sweating, pumped-up jerk next to you in the gym is killing himself. It is a great consolation. Reasonable, regular and sustained exercise will definitely make you feel better and seems likely to extend your life somewhat. One doctor said an hour in the gym may give you an extra hour of life. Of course, if you hate being in the gym, that is no deal at all.

There is some dispute over whether slightly fatter or slightly thinner people live longer. Calorie restrictionists will argue that very thin people – if well nourished – definitely do. And almost everybody will agree that very fat people definitely don't. So, whatever you eat, don't be fat. But in the middle ground it is unclear so don't fret too much either way.

In terms of what you eat, the Mediterranean diet – unsaturated fats, fish, fruit and vegetables – does seem to work

better than the northern European/American – saturated fats,
sugar, red meat etc. Red wine is, happily, good for you. It is
said to resolve the French paradox. The French eat more red
meat than most Mediterraneans but don't seem to die as soon
as they should. Red wine offers the resolution because it
seems to provide some protection against heart attacks and
various other killers including cancer. This may be so, but, on
the other hand, wine contains alcohol and sugars, both
thought to be life-shortening, so, typically, the supplement
industry has found a way of selling just the bit of red wine
that seems to do you good. This is known as Resveratrol. It is
a compound found in the skin of red grapes and is advertised
as 'the French paradox in a bottle'. It is taken by a very high
number of the immortalists I met, most of whom drink little
or no alcohol. It is said to be antioxidant, anti-cancer, and a
phytoestrogen which may help women with the menopause
but may make men impotent, a combination that feels, cruelly, like two sides of the same coin. It has been shown to
extend the lifespan of yeast as well as some worms and fish.
I am suspicious of this for the same reason that I am suspicious of the idea that a vitamin C pill is as good as eating an
orange. In isolating the apparently beneficial essence, we may
be losing something of value.

Other than that, dietary advice is hard to assess. Recent
medical attention has turned to the damage done by low level
but chronic inflammation that kills you in the long run. It is
possible that some foods cause this problem, though it is not
clear which. It is one reason why a low-dose aspirin a day is
almost universally regarded as a good idea. Excessive saturated fats also seem to be generally agreed to be a bad thing.
They are said to lead to plaques forming in the blood vessels
which can kill you via a heart attack or a stroke. There are,
however, still disputes about the link between the formation
of these plaques and dietary cholesterol. Some say the cho-

lesterol levels are entirely genetically determined and dietary levels have no impact; others argue that the plaques are caused by inflammation or even by a viral infection.

The brain is the organ most vulnerable to ageing. It's not really made to last more than a maximum of about a hundred years so, if the above measures get you to that age, you may find yourself without a functioning 'you' to appreciate it. Basically, the brain rots, but on the other hand it benefits even more than the body from exercise. Studies of ageing brains universally show that disciplined cognitive pursuits – chess, crosswords, serious reading, deep thought, almost anything more organised than staring blankly into the middle distance or watching TV game shows – can be maintained at more or less consistently high levels in spite of brain rot. They can also, to some limited extent, help in conditions like Alzheimer's.

There is, finally, one triple recommendation that is given to some medical students by a teacher sceptical of most current attempts to prolong life. 'Be nice,' he says, 'be thin and have daughters.' These are not, strictly speaking, medical recommendations. Rather, they are intended to make the time available to you as pleasant as possible. If you are nice, people will like you and be nice in return. If you are thin, apart from probably being in better condition, you will also acquire respect – studies have shown that fat people are less well respected. And, if you have daughters, they, as opposed to ungrateful sons, will look after you in old age. All of which might lengthen your life but, more likely, it will simply make you more at ease with what you have.

'The utility of living', wrote Michel de Montaigne, 'consists not in the length of days, but in the use of time; a man may have lived long, and yet lived but little.'

Not much more can confidently be said. We may be on the verge of a longevity breakthrough, but if we are then it is startling how little we currently know for certain about how to extend life very much at the moment. Furthermore, even when we appear to know almost everything about diseases that kill us – as in the case of cancer – we remain quite unable to find an effective remedy or prophylactic. Nevertheless, knowledge is advancing on an ever broader front and, if the immortalists are even half right, then we may, indeed, be about to see a sudden change in our prospects. This is, of course, a very big 'if'.

7

Survival Then?

The 'If'

The size of the 'if' is a matter of some dispute. Opinions on when we will achieve significant human life extension and medical immortality vary from never to somewhere between one and three decades. However, the holders of the 'never' view are in a much smaller minority than they were a few years ago. Advances in molecular biology and the more distant possibilities arising from nanotechnology have persuaded most that our medium- to long-term ability to fix the human machine-body is, potentially, unlimited.

Problems remain, the two most intractable being the brain and cancer. The brain is ill-suited to long-term survival and cancer is not so much a disease as a natural if aberrant condition of living cells. The more we discover about it, the more it seems to be embedded in our biology. Removing cell debris in the way that de Grey suggests is spring-cleaning, curing cancer is moving house; it involves a fundamental redesign of the body at a cellular level. If it cannot be done, then the whole project fails as it is statistically certain that cancer would get us all in the end.

Nevertheless, progress is happening in certain areas. In Cambridge in 2005, I saw American scientists demonstrate a procedure whereby they could grow new organs from the patient's own cells. A large number of the doctors present gasped in disbelief. A few months later – in April 2006 – those same scientists, from Wake Forest University Medical School in the US, announced that they had used artificial bladders for children aged from four to nineteen as a way of curing poor bladder function. In the future the same procedure could be used to treat inflammatory diseases and cancer.

The most optimistic boosters of technological advance speak of the Singularity. I shall deal with this in greater detail in my final chapter. But, purely in terms of the speed at which life-extension technology might arrive, it needs to be mentioned here. The Singularity is an idea advanced by Ray Kurzweil and others. It is based on the possibility of continued, exponential growth in the rate of innovation in science and technology. At some point this rate will become so rapid that, in an instant, it will be able to transform the entire world. We cannot predict this moment with any certainty, though it may be linked to the development of effective software emulations of human intelligence by the 2020s. One way or another, if exponential growth is happening and continues to do so, then we can be sure it will happen. All bets and all prophecies will then be off the table. Medical immortality would be upon us in the blinking of an eye.

The Singularity, like the singularity that physicists say lurks at the centre of a black hole, suspends all known laws. It cannot be discussed. So, for the moment, all that can be asked is: what next in the expanding credibility field?

The Mouse

The mouse is the animal that bears the heaviest burden of human hope. This creature has the misfortune to be both sufficiently like us and unlike us to make it the perfect experimental subject. It is like us because it is a mammal and it shares about 85 per cent of our genome or 90 per cent if just genes with known disease links are included. It is unlike us because it does not live as long and so the results of longevity experiments can be more quickly established. Roughly speaking, a twenty-month-old mouse is like a sixty-year-old human in that it is about as likely to suffer from cancer or heart disease. In the wild, mice are unlikely to live as long as one year, though in the benign conditions of the lab they can live much longer. One mouse named Charlie, for example, lived well over four years, purely through careful husbandry.

The mouse, therefore, is the primary target of anti-ageing research. Aubrey de Grey predicts that it will be an extremely long-lived laboratory mouse that will signal to the world the viability of life-extension technology and, in doing so, will transform human politics as people demand government funds be diverted to this kind of research. The problem with this, as de Grey acknowledges, is the size of the required research programme.

'Sounds good, doesn't it?' he has written. 'Good enough to try pretty hard to expedite? How hard? As hard as the United States tried to develop the atomic bomb before the Germans did, say? Surely so. Surely the case for a Manhattan Project to cure ageing is overwhelming.'

The Manhattan Project was one of the most costly research and development projects ever undertaken. If human life extension needs a comparable effort, then anti-ageing funding is going to have to be multiplied many hundreds if not thousands of times from its present levels; it would have to be a

Manhattan Project on a global scale. The first super-long-
lived mouse may trigger that expansion, but for the moment
the task is to create a freakishly old mouse.

To that end, Dave Gobel, an entrepreneurially inclined
benefactor – 'I'm a pathological altruist, I can't help it.' – has
launched the Mprize. This is a prize fund, standing at the
time of writing at around $3.4 million, from which scientists
producing ever more ancient mice are rewarded. It is mod-
elled on the Ansari X Prize, a $10-million fund designed to
encourage private sector innovation in space flight. Its primary award was won by Burt Rutan with his SpaceShipOne,
a design that is to become the basis for Virgin Galactic's
scheme to launch regular space flights for paying customers.

The success of the X Prize made it clear that encouraging
competitive research could stimulate innovation. In the academic world – where most anti-ageing research would have
to take place – this effect could be intense. Academic depart-
ments are seldom well funded and medical research into the
problems of ageing is still relatively poorly financed. There is
also a sense – strongly felt by Gobel – that medical research in
particular seems to be stalled.

'The idea that was capturing me,' he says, 'is that nothing
seems to have been cured since polio . . . I began to ask what
was the reason for that. If you apply the brilliant minds and
all of the schooling of the medical and research community,
was it true that the human body was so intractable that the
only thing you could do was generally make people feel sort
of better until their own body fixed it or was it perhaps an
economic–social phenomenon?'

There are a number of familiar themes here. The polio vaccine was one of the emblematic developments of the fifties.
Its effect was spectacular – the virtual elimination of a very
visible, insidious and harrowing disease, at least in the
developed world. All subsequent medical developments

appear trivial in comparison, usually little more than tinkering with cancer or cardiovascular treatments. And yet, thoughout, there was the consistent background sound of promises being made or of advice being given that might not actually save your life but, then again, might. The successes of the past, not just the polio vaccine but also antibiotics, encouraged the view that radical breakthroughs were possible and likely. When they did not immediately happen, the resulting impatience with normal corporate and academic procedures combined with the rebellion against the strictures of the Cold War resulted in the self-help health and longevity regimes I described in the last chapter. Gobel's Mprize is along the same lines. It is based on the view that the very structure of research was impeding rather than encouraging the development of longevity treatments.

The idea of a prize, says Gobel, is '100 per cent effective' and it does seem to be working. The first Rejuvenation prize from the foundation went to Stephen Spindler at the University of California at Riverside who had used calorie restriction to extend the usual two-year lifespan of his mice to about two and a half years. But the intention is to have a 'laddered series' of prizes to distinguish between different types of achievement. Spindler won by extending the lives of mice with treatment after they had reached middle age. In contrast Andrej Bartke of the Southern Illinois University School of Medicine won the foundation's Longevity prize by knocking out the growth hormone receptor gene of his mice from birth. This meant they were very small but it gave them almost five years of life – equivalent, says Gobel, to creating a 180-year-old human. But the mouse research most favoured by de Grey involves finding ways of clearing toxic waste from the body. This is produced by cellular metabolism and can, in elderly mice or people, account for 20 per cent of the body weight.

Gobel thinks de Grey is right in his optimistic belief that

the mouse breakthrough will occur in the next decade. The reason for Gobel's optimism is that there are now a large number of people who made 'a ton of money' in software and computer technology. They are investing in genome research and that means the necessary funds are becoming available.

Gobel is the kind of calm, groomed, glowing, optimistic, confident, amiable man that only America seems to produce. He was fifty-two when I met him, a babyboomer, but denies that panic at approaching death or at the possibility he may be too old to benefit from life-extension technology is his motivation in running the Mprize.

He says: 'My motivation is a day by day thing. I see people who are an advanced age and, day by day, it would be better if today was as good as yesterday not worse than yesterday. So I'm a one day at a time kind of guy. So I'm not anxious about tomorrow but planning is good . . .'

He has, like most people in the longevity business, a personal health regime. But, unlike most, his centres on an attitude rather than pills. 'My personal health regime is to be with as many friends as I can, to find so much joy in life and to see things in a positive way kind of like Dr Pangloss . . . This is a wonderful place, it truly is. It's important to stop and experience it . . .'

On top of that, he takes the 'regular alphabet' vitamins and, in addition, Bacopa. This is strictly *bacopa monnieri*, an aquatic plant used in ayurvedic – ancient Indian – medicine. It is said to have antioxidant properties, to reduce stress and improve memory and concentration.

Gobel's religious faith leads him to believe there is no after-life for most people. From dust we come and to dust we return. But God can reconstitute human beings if He chooses, like 'rebooting a computer'. Hell, meanwhile, is 'pretty much here'.

The Immortalists' Immortalist

Having repeatedly bumped into him both in cyberspace and the real world, I have yet to form any settled opinion about Aubrey de Grey. I like him, but I don't know whether I believe in him. His appearance, his manner, his schoolboyish enthusiasm and his high intelligence have made him the front man for the entire life-extension movement. Even his Englishness helps. American boosters of dazzling dreams of a high technology future are just too commonplace and are, anyway, always assumed to be on the take; a hippie, monk-ish, beer-loving, extravagantly bearded Englishman, proud of his mastery of the art of sarcasm, is an oddity in these cir-cles. The leader in *Technology Review* that characterised him as a beer-drinking troll with no life indicated, perhaps, that some officer-class Americans would be happier with one of their own leading them into battle. But the resulting backlash suggested that the foot soldiers were happy with pale Aubrey.

Objectively, however, there has to be an issue of belief in de Grey. The attack by twenty-eight scientists published in the journal of the European Molecular Biology Organization and some of the mutterings I have heard cannot be dismissed lightly. The implication is that he just breezily skirts around profound scientific difficulties and hypnotises lay people and would-be believers with his charm and his lucid, plausible eloquence. Furthermore, the mainstream scientists' view is that any such programme of life extension would take decades if not centuries longer than his most optimistic fore-cast of around thirty years. This is primarily because the testing procedures for such radical treatments will have to be extremely rigorous and time-consuming. In any case, they say, the example of cancer should be a warning to all life-extension boosters. We should be able to cure and prevent cancer. But we can't. It may be, as some have suggested, that cancer is the real death clock, a condition so intimately bound up with our life processes that nothing can be done about it. In that context, de Grey is the supreme raiser of false hopes.

De Grey simply believes his critics are too obsessed with their existing procedures and practices to see the oncoming revolution. They are stuck in a conceptual mind trap. He is an engineer. They prefer to learn before they do. He prefers to focus on doing. This is, after all, an emergency. People are dying.

Who knows? But, if the subtext of all these attacks is that he is in any way fraudulent or mad, then I am sure the critics are wrong. For all his courting of the media, there is an innocence about de Grey. He is fired by ambition but not, as far as I can tell, by money. He is driven by conviction and, though odd and obsessed, is as sane as anybody who decides to fling themselves into a single lifelong project.

His method is to isolate the seven well-defined causes of ageing and then to work out how these can be fixed one by one. There is no over-arching theory, simply a narrow focus on what actually happens. The seven causes are not in themselves controversial. In brief, these are his causes of ageing:

1) Cell depletion. Cells are normally replaced, but not always, notably in our brain, heart and muscles. This can be remedied in three ways: exercise to stimulate cell activity, the injection of growth factors to stimulate division and the introduction of fresh cells. The latter is the most radical and so-far untested idea. It involves the use of stem-cell technology.

2) Cell excess. As we age, certain cells increase in number. These are fat cells, senescent cells that accumulate primarily in cartilage and certain types of immune cells. The latter are, in effect, an overreaction by the body to certain types of infection. This unbalances the immune

system. The solution may involve persuading certain cells to commit suicide or using the immune system to kill them.

3) Mutations in the chromosome. Our DNA is well protected and most mutations are harmless. Cancer, however, kills on the basis of a single mutation in a single cell. So the problem is not to attack mutations as such, simply to attack cancer. De Grey's preferred strategy is WILT – Whole-body Interdiction of Lengthening of Telomeres. This is complex and highly controversial but de Grey insists we are already close to achieving it in mice.

4) Mitochondrial mutations. Mitochondria are the fuel sources of the cell and they contain the only DNA in the body outside the nucleus. Unfortunately, it is more prone to mutation and so, with age, mitochondrial function declines. De Grey wants to transfer the DNA for the thirteen genes on mitochondrial DNA into the nucleus where they will be better protected.

5) Cells break down large molecules and some of the debris from this process builds up within the cell. Regularly dividing cells dilute this but non-dividing cells become increasingly clogged. This causes atherosclerosis, degeneration of the brain and blindness. De Grey wants to give the cells extra enzymes to break down the most intractable junk.

6) Debris outside the cells. The worst example is amyloid which forms plaques inside the brain – this happens to everybody but most disastrously in Alzheimer's patients. Vaccination to stimulate the immune system to engulf this material is the current most likely solution.

7) Crosslinks. With age, proteins outside the cell start to form crosslinks that stiffen tissue and, in the case of the eyes, renders it opaque. This may be simply solved with

a drug that dissolves these links without damaging sur-
rounding tissue. Some are now in development.

'We have a pretty good idea how to fix all of them,' says de
Grey, 'and some of the fixes are in clinical trials. But the
point is we don't have to fix all of them completely.'

Cellular junk, for example, has no effect until it passes a
certain point. This seems to happen when people are aged
about thirty. If, therefore, the junk can be reduced to the
levels before this started to happen, the problem is contained.
The difficult problem of eliminating all cellular junk is thus
reduced to the simpler one of just eliminating some of it.

Unlike most immortalists, the forty-one-year-old de Grey
does not pursue a punishing survival regime: 'I'm very lucky
genetically, I eat and drink more or less what I want and I
don't even do all that much exercise, yet I have maintained an
absolutely constant weight since I was seventeen ... My
mother lives in Chelsea and I live in Cambridge. I know how
long it takes me to cycle from King's Cross to my mother's
house. It's spot on what it was when I was eighteen.'

It's Easy to Die

De Grey is the current prophet of life extension, his still active
predecessor – whom he admires effusively – is Michael West.
Yet West is almost the opposite of de Grey. He is entrepre-
neurial and clever though not in the extravagantly
demonstrative way of de Grey. Rather, he delivers his message
with the honed simplicity of a chief executive. He is the chair-
man and chief scientific officer of Advanced Cell Technology
(ACT) and he was the founder of the Geron Corporation. His
Americanness is as clear and defined as is de Grey's
Englishness.

This Americanness also extends to a religiosity which is

wholly absent from de Grey. In his book *The Immortal Cell*, he describes his obsession with and his attempts to make sense of Christianity. He writes: 'The Bible absorbed me as a sponge absorbs a drop of water. What a glorious solution to the problem of mortality. This, I realized, was the greatest force people feel drawing them to religion. It was a magnificent story of love conquering death.'

And he quotes William James: 'Religion in fact, for the great majority of our own race *means* immortality, and nothing else. God is the producer of immortality.'

But he wanted proof and, ultimately, the Bible offers only faith. He spent five years 'looking to carefully document the fingerprints of the creator in the world of nature'. Finally, however, he accepted the theory of evolution, that people are part of nature and then discovered that 'I had lost my moorings.' And then his father died.

'I realized that it was simply not in my nature to accept death or be defeated by it. The call wasn't even a close one. I could never again resign myself to laying my loved ones down in the grave.'

He sees this visionary conversion as a rejection of religion, but it doesn't sound like it. He speaks of his 'mission' and his public speeches are replete with prophetic force. Even his interpretation of the science of immortality has a salvational ring. He regards with 'distaste' the immortal germ line, from the perspective of which the human body is merely a disposable vehicle.

The germ line view is an offence against individuality, the supreme American virtue. How far this is all just rhetoric to further his business causes I cannot say. Some seem to mistrust him. When, early in this decade, ACT announced the first known cloning of a human embryo just at the time George Bush was restricting the use of embyros West was widely trashed by fellow scientists.

Geneticist Lee Silver said he just wanted to be 'the Bill Gates of cloning' and a Nobel prizewinning microbiologist said the announcement had 'aggravated the debate and has the potential to drive important scientific research off-shore'. The bioethicist Arthur Caplan points out that West has: 'religious and theological inspirations. But he also comes across as a fire-breathing, secular businessman.' And the bio-conservative political magazine *The Weekly Standard* compared him to Osama bin Laden in that both terrorism and cloning pose 'grave threats to a dignified human future'.

West's business adventures are well known, his scientific significance less so. His method is pragmatic, like de Grey's, but he does not employ a strict engineering approach. Rather, he simply attacks two very general areas. One is stem cells. Stem cells are undifferentiated. They are able to become any cell in the body. They could, in theory, be used to repair diseased tissue – say, the brain in Parkinson's disease patients – or grow new organs that would not be rejected. At the moment, they look like one of the key tools in life-extension technology, but it is not yet clear how this will be done across the broad spectrum of human pathology. Conceptually, their significance is immense. In effect, they give us access to the immortality of the germ line and offer the possibility of transferring that immortality to the somatic cells.

It ought to be said that this link between the immortality of the germ line and of the whole organism is regarded with scepticism by many scientists. Robert Weinberg of the Massachusetts Institute of Technology spoke for them all when he attacked the basis of the work of Geron, West's original company. Weinberg is a cancer specialist so his awareness of the intractability of that condition evidently plays a part in his scepticism: 'There has been the implication that cellular immortalization will translate in some way to lengthening – if not greatly extending – the life span of an organism. This is irrational. But that irrationality has been exploited by companies like Geron . . .'

West's second key area of research is into telomeres. A telomere is a length of DNA at the end of each chromosome that consists simply of repetitive sequences of nucleotide bases. This seems to act as a buffer to prevent the chromosome being damaged in the replication process. In achieving this, however, the telomere progressively shortens so that the telomeres of older people are shorter than those of younger. Conceivably, therefore, preserving the telomeres could halt some of the effects of ageing. It has certainly done so in some animal models in which the enzyme telomerase has been used to extend the telomeres. It is unclear whether it would work in humans. The complication may be that extending the telomeres could result in the production of tumours. Indeed, de Grey's WILT strategy on cancer is aimed precisely at stopping this happening.

Again, it is hard to know what to make of West. He is a hard-sell businessman and a born-again believer in medical life extension as opposed to the immortality offered by conventional faith. At the heart of his drive is his strong sense that immortality exists in the form of the germ cells. He says: 'I don't know the answers to the big questions . . . what I do know is that you and I are made from cells that have an immortal legacy all the way back to the origins of life.'

When I met him and conducted a breathless interview at Cambridge, he seemed to speak partly on autopilot and partly as a hot gospeller. He is, in some ways, even more optimistic than de Grey, seeing some major applications of what he calls 'regenerative medicine' within a decade. When I asked him if he'd take an immortality pill, it was as if I'd asked the Pope if he believed in God.

'Oh sure. We can always die, it's easy to die and be free of debilitating disease is I think the foundation. We can get tired of life, when life gets boring, it's easy to die. . . . Not having the choice is part of it and the suffering that is inherent. People in my mind respond to grief and terminal illness with resignation.'

Everything about West revolves around this rejection of resignation, this fierce and very American conviction that saving the individual is, in the end, all that matters.

The Immortal Flies

There is one further important hint that we may not be as inevitably mortal as we once thought. This springs from a bizarre, statistical finding about the ageing and death of fruit flies and it is related to Kirkwood's disposable soma theory. Essentially, we seem to have discovered that, beyond a certain point, old fruit flies stop ageing.

The leading proponent of this view is Michael Rose of the University of California at Irving. He has studied the way death rates in fruit flies simply seem to level off. This is not to say they don't die, of course, by a certain time they are so frail that something will kill them all. But it is to say that, day by day, they do not become more *likely* to die. Since increased likelihood of dying is the most generally accepted definition of ageing, this means the flies have, in fact, ceased to age.

The relationship to Kirkwood's theory is that there may come a point where the antagonistic effect of genes ceases. Evolutionary pressures cease and nature leaves the old fly to die of whatever happens to come along.

A chart of the death rates of fruit flies shows a familiar rise as they grow older followed by a very unfamiliar plateau at which they seem to become 'biologically immortal'. The implication of Rose's work is that, if such a condition as biological immortality exists, then we could move this plateau down the chart, making the flies immortal at earlier ages. If this could be done, then the 'immortal' flies would be in much better condition and less likely to die from sheer frailty. Ultimately, we could arrange for the plateau to occur before any ageing happened at all, at which point the flies would be fully medically immortal.

This is speculative and many, de Grey included, are sceptical, seeing the whole idea as a statistical artefact. But, like so many other anti-death ideas, it is in the air, firing the enthusiasm of the immortalists.

Without a Stitch or Scar

Molecular biology – which includes, among many other things, stem-cell research – is seen as the next step in the treatment of disease. But it is only, in Ray Kurzweil's terms, the first bridge to the future. The second is nanotechnology, an almost open-ended realm of possibilities constructed on the possibility of molecular-sized machines.

'Reaching an era with advanced cell repair machines', wrote Eric Drexler, 'seems the key to long life and health, because almost all physical problems will then be curable.'

It was Drexler's book *Engines of Creation* that in the late eighties generated widespread interest in nanotechnology and launched a speculative boom. Like cryonics, nanotechnology seems infinite in its promise. Human immortality is almost a by-product of its explosion of possibilities.

A nanometre is one billionth of a metre. It is the measure of atoms and molecules. If we can work at this scale – and, to a limited extent, we already can – then we are potentially in control of all matter. We will not be inhibited by working with materials but, rather, with their ultimate constituents. And we will do so through mechanical proxies. Nanotechnology involves the building of molecular-sized machines – sometimes called nanobots – that would reassemble, rearrange and repair matter atom by atom.

Cryonicists love nanotechnology. At a stroke it seems to dispel all scepticism about their freezing procedures. The capability of nanobots could be such that, no matter what damage had been done during the processes of disease, dying and freezing, the body could be rebuilt one molecule at a time. In Drexler's book there is a dramatic, almost dream-like account of the revival of a frozen patient: 'Now the machines pump in a milky fluid containing trillions of devices that enter cells and remove the glassy protectant. Molecule by molecule . . . Outside the body, the repair system has grown fresh blood from the patient's own cells . . . the repair system closes the opening in the chest, joining tissue to tissue without a stitch or a scar.'

In the living, nanotechnology could achieve what Robert Freitas of the Institute for Molecular Manufacturing calls 'dechronification', removing the effects of age on the body. Injected nanobots would enter each cell in the body and clean out debris and toxins – this could either be done continuously or annually – they would correct any damage to DNA and they would repair any damaged structures, like mitochondria, within the cells.

Nanotechnology might rebuild our entire bodies, dispensing with haphazardly designed and often inefficient substances like blood and replacing it with, say, a fluid that pumps itself, removing the need for a heart, and acquires its own energy source, removing the need for breathing.

In the brain, nanobots will create what Kurzweil calls 'a hybrid of both biological and nonbiological intelligence'. Both the number and speed of connections would be massively increased.

'This will enable you,' wrote Kurzweil, 'to profoundly expand your pattern recognition, cognitive, and emotional capacities as well as provide intimate connection to powerful new forms of nonbiological thinking. You will also have the means for direct high bandwidth communication to the Internet and other people from your brain.'

Telepathy would become a clear reality through a technology to the wireless computer systems we have today. Another dream of the hunters of the white crow will have been realised.

Machine Salvation

With the aid of nanobots, the body moves towards the condition of the eternally fixable machine. The opposite development may also save us – the machine may move towards us.

Artificial intelligence (AI) has, along with space exploration, been one of the great disappointments of contemporary technology. Just as fifty years ago we were promised planetary if not interstellar exploration in the near future, so we were promised intelligent machines. Neither has happened and both, in some ways, have appeared to go backwards. Perhaps both are beyond us.

Any such sentiment would, of course, be heresy to the technophile heroes of this book. For them, artificial intelligence is imminent. It will contribute to the immortalist cause either by applying its own enhanced brain to the problems involved or by providing us with an opportunity to down (up?) load ourselves into a machine with a capability of backing ourselves up like a computer programme. The pursuit of AI runs in parallel with the medical effort.

Like nanotechnology, there is a bracing vastness about the AI future. As Nick Bostrom has said, this would be the last machine human beings would ever have to make. Once we had created this super-intelligence, it would be able to do more things far better than we ever could. Moreover, it would tend to evolve away from us by designing ever-superior versions of itself. We couldn't even talk to it in any meaningful way as, beyond a certain point, it would not be able to explain its projects and motives in any terms we could understand – just as we could not currently explain ourselves to a chimpanzee. This is an enormous risk, of course, and AI researcher Hugo de Garis has compared his own position to that of nuclear physicists of the 1930s and 1940s. They knew they were heading towards a bomb just as he knows he is heading towards a machine that might simply sweep us aside – or ensure our immortality.

The Omega Point

The final and perhaps the most bizarre way we may be saved from oblivion is the Omega Point Theory, a term coined by the strange, occasionally comprehensible French Jesuit theologian Pierre Teilhard de Chardin. Chardin followed Hegel in seeing history as the unfolding of spirit. But he went much further in his belief in the evolution of the 'noosphere' – the realm of consciousness – towards a final Omega Point at which the maximum level of consciousness in the cosmos would have been attained.

The idea was taken up by Frank Tipler, a physicist at Tulane University. He produced his version of the Omega Point Theory in his book *The Physics of Immortality: Modern Cosmology, God and the Resurrection of the Dead* (1994). Tipler argued that there was scientific basis for a Chardinian cosmic climax. Tipler's importance lies in the very fact that he put such an argument. Ever since quantum theory and relativity revealed a much stranger universe than had been thought, there has been intense speculation about the meaning of what we have discovered. Specifically, in writers like Fritjof Capra and Dana Zohar, there have been attempts to relate the insights of quantum theory directly to the human realm, often through parallels with eastern religious thought. These represented a longing to bring science back into the human fold, in effect, to offset the catastrophic effects its success appeared to have had in diminishing the claims of spirituality. Tipler's claim, however, is much more specific. He is saying that science has revealed our true immortal destiny, that in fact it has proved religion to be true.

'I have been forced into these conclusions', he writes, 'by the inexorable logic of my own special branch of physics.'

His argument is based on a radical and much more temporally distant version of the Singularity. Ultimately, he argues, scientific and technological progress will enable us to take control of the entire universe. At the Omega Point – the moment in the future which he identifies with God – the universe will have become a single, gigantic artificial intelligence. But some time before this point, possibly only a few thousand years in the future, some such machine will be capable of running perfect simulations of every life form that has ever existed, ourselves included.

But the point about these simulations is that they will not really be simulations. Rather, they will be exact recreations of the quantum conditions of the original individual. I, as I am now, therefore, will be reawoken at – possibly the correct word is 'in' – the Omega Point with all my memories and sense of self intact. This will be heaven and it will be a very anthropocentric heaven, though with overtones of the virtual world evoked in the *Matrix* series of films. For, in order to duplicate the individual, we would have also to duplicate his environment. In fact: 'Since humans also interact with their inanimate environment, to get the exact quantum state, it might even be necessary to replicate the entire visible universe.'

This, it seems to me, could already have happened and we are living in this universal simulation. But, at least, if it has we are all truly immortal because, though the universe may well be in the last stages of its final collapse, the supreme AI will have also mastered time. This will enable our new selves to last forever, whatever fate befalls the material cosmos.

Physicists may agree or, more often, disagree with the science behind such a claim. The rest of us need only notice that the claim has been made. In this book, Tipler becomes the heir to the tradition of the psychical researchers of the nineteenth century – men like Myers, Lodge and Crookes. Like them, he attempts to use the tools of science to show that the scientific project thus far has been flawed. In its narrow focus on the experimental method, it has failed to see the big picture, failed to realise that the religion it appeared to be disproving was, in fact, re-emerging from within its discoveries. The black crow project was founded upon an illusion; in reality, all the crows were white.

Anton Chekhov

The most striking thing about these possible solutions to the problem of death is their number and variety. Death is being attacked on many fronts. Furthermore, even within these fronts, there are an enormous number of smaller fronts. The list I have given is a radical distillation of current life-extension science. I know of many more research approaches. There will be even more of which I am entirely ignorant. One might say that the whole of medical science is part of this project. But, of course, it is only those areas in which scientists are explicit about their goal of extending life indefinitely that are truly relevant because only in those areas do we hear the rhetoric and reasoning behind such an aspiration.

Confronted with this variety, sceptics will be reminded of

the dry warning of Anton Chekhov – that if there are many cures for a disease, then you can sure there is no cure. The very fact that we are thrashing around with such abandon puts us in the position of those hapless doctors in *Madame Bovary* or *The Death of Ivan Ilyich* who use intense activity to disguise their ignorance.

The answer to that, of course, is that it is precisely this multi-front assault that is most likely to lead to success, not least because success in the form of a treatment is likely to be complex and to involve many different types of therapy. There is, at the moment, no likelihood of one simple fix for the human body.

But now even 'deathists' like Leon Kass acknowledge that we must consider the future in the light of the possibility that the immortalists might, indeed, come up with something. And so it is at last time to ask the same question as Sadie Sturdivant, the sad and baffled friend of Henrietta Lacks, the woman who attained a strange, cellular immortality after her death from cancer. 'What it really mean?' asked Sadie.

8

Survival. But?

Some Transhumanists

Outside the conference hall in Atlanta, a strange, awkward-looking young man had been watching me as I conducted interviews at a low coffee table. He would sidle slowly past, his eyes fixed on me. If I turned to face him, he would smile encouragingly as if prompting me to say something. He had not been on my list of interviewees, but he plainly thought he ought to be. After a time, I succumbed, partly because his behaviour had begun to spook me and partly because anybody so determined to be interviewed might just have something to say.

I was right on both counts. He was spooky and he did have something interesting to say. The spookiness was three-fold. First, there was his manner of amused, nervous detachment from the conversation as if he was having some difficulty in engaging at my level. He had the air of a precocious schoolboy. The second element of spookiness arose from the two young men who joined us. Both laughed knowingly and nodded wisely at his every remark; they also nodded at the questions I asked, but with an air of pity. The third spooky thing lay in what he thought.

Eliezer Yudkowsky was then twenty-six and was already signed up to the Cryonics Institute in Michigan. Both he and his admirers say he is a genius. His genius was inspired by a paper written by the mathematician and science-fiction author Vernon Vinge and delivered to a symposium in 1993. At the heart of this paper was the concept of the Singularity, an idea Vinge had in part derived from a reported remark made in the 1950s by the great mathematician and computer scientist John von Neumann.

'One conversation centred', ran Stan Ulam's recollection of the conversation, 'on the ever accelerating progress of technology and changes in the mode of human life, which gives the appearance of approaching some essential singularity in the history of the race beyond which human affairs, as we know them, could not continue.'

It is not clear what von Neumann meant, but two important ideas are present. First, there is the ever-increasing rate of technological progress. This was later to be the basis of Moore's law. This is not, in fact, a law at all but a simple observation made by Gordon Moore, co-founder of Intel. This stated that computing power – in terms of the complexity of an integrated circuit or chip – doubled every eighteen months. The concept of such inevitable law-like progress lay behind von Neumann's Singularity which may be said to be a generalisation of Moore's law.

Secondly, there is the idea of a point at which this acceleration results in a complete change in human affairs. As in physics, where what is called a singularity at the heart of a black hole is the point at which all known laws cease to apply, so in the human world the Singularity will mark the point at which all previous categories of thought and action will be rendered invalid.

Vinge's paper, however, pursued a more precise implication of the idea:

I argue in this paper that we are on the edge of change comparable to the rise of human life on Earth. The precise cause of this change is the imminent creation by technology of entities with greater than human intelligence. There are several means by which science may achieve this breakthrough (and this is another reason for having confidence that the event will occur):

- There may be developed computers that are 'awake' and superhumanly intelligent. (To date, there has been much controversy as to whether we can create human equivalence in a machine. But if the answer is 'yes, we can', then there is little doubt that beings more intelligent can be constructed shortly thereafter.)
- Large computer networks (and their associated users) may 'wake up' as a superhumanly intelligent entity.
- Computer/human interfaces may become so intimate that users may reasonably be considered superhumanly intelligent.
- Biological science may provide the means to improve natural human intellect.

The reason superhuman artifical intelligence becomes the Singularity is that at that point new and, to us, unimaginable thoughts will be thought. We shall have crossed the threshold into the black hole.

'From the human point of view,' said Vinge, 'this change will be a throwing away of all the previous rules, perhaps in the blink of an eye, an exponential runaway beyond any hope of control.'

This 'blink of an eye' transfiguration strangely echoes the

rapture of American fundamentalism when the true believers will be removed from their earthly existence. And, indeed, prophets of the Singularity do often stress the suddenness and totality of the effect. Ray Kurzweil also stresses its imminence: 'I set the date for the Singularity – representing a profound and disruptive transformation in human capability – as 2045.'

The rapture, however, is plainly an expression of goodness; there is nothing necessarily good about the Singularity. Even Kurzweil acknowledges this – 'Although neither utopian nor dystopian, this epoch will transform the concepts we rely on to give meaning to our lives, from our business models to the cycle of human life, including death itself.'

But is this desirable? The Singularity, in transforming all human categories, also transforms those of good and bad *for us*. There can be no guarantee that any such super-intelligence would have the slightest interest in doing anything that might benefit humans. Indeed, it might come to regard us as little more than belligerent, dirty, stupid inconveniences. Given such a huge risk, it is difficult to imagine what incentive humans could possibly have in working towards the Singularity. Enter Eliezer Yudkowsky.

In 2000, Yudkowsky became one of the three co-founders of the Singularity Institute for Artificial Intelligence in Palo Alto, California, the heart of Silicon Valley. It was 'a non-profit research think tank and public interest institute for the study and advancement of beneficial artificial intelligence and ethical cognitive enhancement'. The following year Yudkowsky produced his own paper entitled 'Creating Friendly AI. 1.0: The Analysis and Design of Benevolent Goal Architectures'. The paper outlined a way of ensuring that the artificial super-intelligence would be friendly. It was enthusiastically received. The details of the argument are less important than the goal which was simply to prevent the sci-fi scenario in which the machines took over and abolished or enslaved us.

There are two ways in which such a machine would be significant for the project of human immortality. It would accelerate medical research into the problems of ageing and dying. Instead of waiting decades or centuries for the creation of nano-machines that would continually remake our bodies, we could have them at once. Or the machine would offer us the opportunity of becoming machines ourselves, uploading our consciousness into computers and thus completely transcending our biological condition. Yudkowsky is personally more keen on the first benefit as he sees uploading as 'a rather difficult technical task to pull off safely, gracefully, reliably'.

He is in a hurry because he thinks, along with Kurzweil, that the Singularity may be near and he wants to be part of what he has no doubt will be 'the most important event to come along in the last few million years or, hey, why not ever?'

His argument for his own immortality is simply that, in any given week, he wants to live one more week and that will always be the case.

'I want to live one more week and then I will still want to live one more week. I haven't driven a motorcycle, I haven't gone hang-gliding, I haven't studied Riemann's Hypothesis or basic physics. By the time I've done all of those things, I'm sure I'll have wandered across ever more things.'

Keeping the machine good from the moment of its conception is essential.

'After something has already gone wrong, if it was smarter than you, you'd be screwed.'

It is the smartness that renders Isaac Asimov's celebrated Laws of Robotics obsolete. A truly smart and independent-minded machine might simply decide these laws were wrong or inappropriate by way of reasoning processes that we, being less smart, cannot imagine in advance; it would then be free to exterminate us, which, growing smarter by the minute, it would find extremely easy. The goal of the Singularity Institute is to define ways of designing a machine that would make such anti-human malevolence impossible. Yudkowsky uses a brief thought experiment to explain how this might be done.

'Are you likely', he asks, 'to take a pill that makes you want to kill babies?'

The machine can repeatedly reprogramme itself; the trick, therefore, is to set moral limits to these transformations so that taking a pill to kill babies would be as inconceivable to it as it would be to me. But is killing babies that inconceivable to me? It certainly isn't to other members of my species. Human beings kill babies with remarkable frequency.

'The most natural thing of all for humans', says Max More, 'is to change nature.'

More is a pale, balding, red-haired man, who speaks rather breathlessly, snatching at each clause as if with some kind of difficulty. He was forty-one when we met and he would not tell me his original surname. I later discovered it was O'Connor. He changed it to More because, he says, 'I want more.' Having set up the first cryonics organisation in the UK, he moved from Britain to America in 1987 to work on his PhD in philosophy at the University of Southern California. In 1991 he founded the Extropy Institute, which, like the Singularity Institute, is inspired by the conviction that technology is increasingly rapidly driving changes in the human condition. Extropy is a neologism which implies the opposite of entropy, though More prefers to say it is a metaphor for 'increasing order and information, all the good things in life . . .'

'I've always been driven by this idea that humanity is not a final state, we can keep evolving and improving and I think if we get too stuck in what we are and our nature, it doesn't change. I think now more and more people are realising that things are changing and maybe faster than you might expect though not as fast as some of us would hope.'

More defines extropy as 'an evolving framework of values and standards for continuously improving the human condition'. It has seven principles, which are more or less self-explanatory: perpetual progress, self-transformation, practical optimism, intelligent technology, open society, self direction and rational thinking. It is not, he insists, an ideology.

'I don't believe I have the best plan for everybody in the universe and this is what we ought to do in the future. . . . I'm much more of the Enlightenment view that I want to give people the scientific and technological freedom to be how we want to be ourselves rather than to restrain people.'

The key freedom, the freedom that makes all others possible, is, of course, freedom from death.

'I'd like to have the option to live for as long as I wanted. It doesn't mean I want to live forever because I don't know that, I can't speak for my future. Maybe 20,000 years from now I might decide that's sufficient, I don't know. But all I know is right now I see no reason to die just because nature says it is time to. That programme is completely arbitrary, it has no special status at all. There's no reason to accept it.'

More started taking vitamins at the age of twelve. He continues to do so, combining them with a good diet, exercise and stress reduction. He also has a personal vitamin formula prescribed for him by the Kronos Longevity Research Institute in Phoenix. Like everybody else involved with this cause, he wants to be around to benefit from its triumphant vindication.

He has become one of the primary advocates of life-extension research. He is a polemicist, fighting a battle against those who would resist or attempt to regulate this technology. His latest arguments centre on the Proactionary Principle, constructed in opposition to the Precautionary Principle. The latter argues for the avoidance of risk as far as possible; the former for the acceptance of a degree of risk on the basis that potential rewards are enormous. The Extropy Institute website gives a ringing call to proactionary arms: '. . . Let a thousand flowers bloom! By all means, inspect the flowers for signs of infestation and weed as necessary. But don't cut off the hands of those who spread the seeds of the future.'

In Oxford, I met Nick Bostrom, then a thirty-one-year-old philosopher, director of the Oxford Future of Humanity Institute and co-founder of the World Transhumanist Association. An amiable, but very precise man, he is perhaps the leading transhumanist thinker in the world. He is certainly among the clearest.

'For as long as I can remember it seemed clear to me that the most decisive factor in determining the future of humankind would be new technological developments that could radically change . . . human biology, human capacities.'

All previous futuristic dreams have been scuppered by one source of fatal error. People. Projects of the left – socialism and communism – of the right – Nazism and fascism – and of the religious – almost all major faiths have a millennarian wing, notably in our time the American Christian and Islamic fundamentalists – have all foundered, or will founder, because people did not live up to the visions of their leaders. So utopians can't fix people by reorganising externalities like politics and society; they must fix the internalities, how people feel and think, what they are, when they die. Hence transhumanism, perhaps the only area left in which rational thought can still decently claim to be world-transforming.

'If I wanted to make some positive difference in the world,'

says Bostrom, 'this would be the area with the greatest lever-
age . . . It's an extension of humanism. It has its roots in
secular humanism and it shares a lot of its principles with
humanism – the idea that human beings are relying on their
own powers rather than in deference to supernatural intervention. It's about rational thinking and democracy and so
forth, improving the human condition . . .

'There is the crucial difference in that rather than imposing
some big, grand solutions across the board like past utopian
dreamers, transhumanists just want to provide people with
these options . . .'

Not dying is one crucial option. Bostrom, like many others,
extrapolates our existing high estimation of the value of
human life to argue for a massive and radical research programme aimed at extending lives indefinitely. His very
striking contribution to the immortalist cause is *The Fable of
the Dragon Tyrant*.This is a fairy story about an evil dragon
that ruled over an apparently helpless people. It is virtually a
sacred text among immortalists.

> It demanded from humankind a blood-curdling tribute: to
> satisfy its enormous appetite, ten thousand men and
> women had to be delivered every evening at the onset of
> dark to the foot of the mountain where the dragon-tyrant
> lived. Sometimes the dragon would devour these unfortu-
> nate souls upon arrival; sometimes again it would lock
> them up in the mountain where they would wither away
> for months or years before eventually being consumed.

Everybody ends up being consumed by the dragon which
is, of course, death. Religions spring up to justify the slaughter or to console people with the prospect of a life after they
have been devoured. But one prophet rose up to say that, one
day, people would find a way to slay the dragon. Finally, the

technology becomes available and, after much argument and great resistance from the religious types – 'The phrases were so eloquent that it was hard to resist the feeling that some deep thoughts must lurk behind them, although nobody could quite grasp what they were.' – a missile is launched that kills the dragon. The king is at first distraught, wondering why this had not been done years before, saving millions of lives. But finally he addresses the people: 'My dear friends, we have come a long way ... yet our journey has only just begun. Our species is young on this planet. Today we are like children again. The future lies open before us ...'

Slaying the dragon tyrant – fixing the human body – is only the beginning. Phase two is fixing the human soul.

Boredom

The first part of the philosophical case against the transhumanist and immortalist positions is that it is perilous to meddle with human nature and that death is an essential aspect of our humanity; the second, much more complex and profound part is the argument about the endless life and boredom.

Francis Fukuyama and Leon Kass, a bioethicist at the University of Chicago and presidential adviser, support the human-nature case. It is Kass's lecture – 'L'Chaim and its Limits: Why Not Immortality?', delivered in Jerusalem in 2000 – that most lucidly and eloquently puts this case against the immortalists and which has inspired their most energetic and occasionally angry rebuttals. Since the lecture is a brilliant summary of the anti-immortalist position and is generally understood as such, I shall summarise it at some length.

Kass acknowledges possible external dangers of immortality like the disruption of social order, the creation of rank injustices if some can afford it and others can't and so on. But his primary concern is with the internal dangers, with the threats to the soul.

'Conquering death', he says, 'is not something that we can try for a while and then decide whether the results are better or worse – according to, God only knows, what standard. On the contrary, this is a question in which our very humanity is at stake . . .'

Kass suggests four ways in which immortality will be bad for our souls. It will diminish our interest and engagement in life, it will compromise our seriousness and our aspirations, it will destroy beauty and love and it will remove the possibilities of virtue and moral excellence. All of these things are defined by the knowledge of our own deaths. Without them, it is difficult to know who we would be, how we would evaluate anything. Immortality, says Kass, would be 'a kind of oblivion – like death itself'. Kass knows that these arguments will seem absurd to contemporary imaginations suffused with the belief in the self, with the L'Oréal 'Because you're worth it!' culture. Kass says: 'Moreover, though some cultures – such as the Eskimo – can instruct and moderate somewhat the lust for life, liberal Western society gives it free rein, beginning with a political philosophy founded on a fear of violent death, and reaching to our current cults of youth and novelty, the cosmetic replastering of the wrinkles of age, and the widespread anxiety about disease and survival.'

But haven't humans always longed for immortality? Shouldn't this also be seen as a defining aspect of human nature? Kass's answer is that religious immortality occurs in a different plane, in a different life.

What is it that we lack and long for, but cannot reach? One possibility is completion in another person. For example, Plato's Aristophanes says we seek wholeness through complete and permanent bodily and psychic union with a unique human being whom we love, our 'missing other half'. Plato's Socrates, in contrast, says it is rather wholeness through wisdom, through comprehensive knowledge of the beautiful truth about the whole, that which philosophy seeks but can never attain. Yet again, biblical religion says we seek wholeness through dwelling in God's presence, love, and redemption – a restoration of innocent wholeheartedness lost in the Garden of Eden. But, please note, these . . . all agree on this crucial point: man longs not so much for deathlessness as for wholeness, wisdom, goodness, and godliness – longings that cannot be satisfied fully in our embodied earthly life, the only life, by natural reason, we know we have. Hence the attractiveness of any prospect or promise of a different and thereby fulfilling life hereafter. The decisive inference is clear: none of these longings can be answered by prolonging earthly life. Not even an unlimited amount of 'more of the same' will satisfy our deepest aspirations.

The Jewish toast – *L'Chaim*, To Life – is interpreted by Kass as an exclamation in honour of life as a whole, not the individual life, and life as a whole includes dying and being born. And, if it did not, it would be a smaller, shrunken thing, an object barely worthy of a toast.

Two important modern philosophers have produced essays advancing parallel but more sophisticated arguments. Both start from the Roman philosopher and poet Lucretius, who argued that fear of death was irrational because we do not fear or regret or suffer as a result of our non-existence before birth, why then should our non-existence after death be viewed any differently?

Thomas Nagel takes on Lucretius by asking himself the question: is it a bad thing to die? He argues that there is no positive evil in the state of death itself, rather there is a negative evil in the loss of all the activities – the goods – of life: 'If we are to make sense of the view that to die is bad, it must be on the grounds that life is good and death is the corresponding deprivation or loss, bad not because of any positive features but because of the desirability of what it removes.'

The problem with seeing death as a loss is that it does not seem so to the dead person because he no longer exists. But Nagel argues that a misfortune does not require the knowledge of the victim. To be betrayed is absolutely bad whether one knows about it or not. So to have lost the goods of life by dying can be seen as a misfortune that has happened to the dead person.

Nagel does not go on to say in this essay that immortality would, therefore, be a good thing, but the implication is there. Bernard Williams – starting from a combination of Lucretius, Nagel and Karel Capek's play *The Makropulos Case* about a woman who has attained immortality – produces a strong argument against immortality as in any way desirable and he echoes Kass's point about immortality as oblivion when he writes, 'an endless life would be a meaningless one'. *The Makropulos Case* is the key to his argument. The heroine has had a headache for 200 years and is simply bored with her eternal life. In her mind, mere mortals have become little more than passing shadows:

> I don't know. Everything is so dull, empty and ordinary –
> Are you all there? It seems as if you were not – as if you
> were things or shadows. What do you want me to do? . . .
> No, it doesn't matter. It's all the same, whether you're here
> or not. And you make such a fuss over each little death.
> You are queer . . .

For Williams, boredom is the problem. This has led to his

argument being rejected out of hand by the immortalists; indeed, their version of Williams has become a fairly consistent strawman in immortalist writings. How could anybody be bored, they exclaim, when there is so much to learn, so much to do? But this is wilfully to miss Williams's real argument, an argument captured by the novelist Milan Kundera. 'What is unbearable in life', he wrote in his novel *Immortality*, 'is not *being* but *being one's self*.'

I have never wished, I do not wish and I am confident I shall never wish to learn how to ski, to speak Wolof or to become an adept mathematician. I have no objection to other people doing these things, but they don't suit me. Of course, I could, one day, change my mind and reluctantly decide to ski, but that is beside the point. What matters is simply that I have a particular character with particular dispositions. If somebody came along and gave me an injection that changed all those dispositions, then, fair enough, but I would have ceased being me. Given an eternity or just one thousand years, I could indeed learn mathematics, but to do so would still bore me.

Or, to put it another way, holidays don't work as they should because, when I get there, I am still me. It is not that I cannot escape the contingencies of my daily life – stress at work, hassles at home – rather, it is that I cannot escape my personality, its dispositions and its entire posture towards the world. I am seeking a holiday from myself, but it is the one thing I, by definition, cannot have. And, if I can never have such a holiday, then I am going to grow bored with myself, bored to death.

Character is Williams's decisive concept in this argument. If we want to live forever, we must avoid boredom. That means always having something to absorb you. If you had no character, you were simply an infinitely voracious intellect, then that might be possible. But no such human being is imaginable. In the end, it is always the same self doing these things and so nothing new and absorbing can ever, beyond a certain point, happen.

'I would eventually', observes Williams, 'have had altogether too much of myself.' Or, as another philosopher, Roger Scruton put it to me, 'You would extend the life of the body beyond the interest the soul would have in inhabiting it.'

This deathist position is obviously rejected by immortalists. They say that we could have successive selves through the course of an extended life. The deathists respond, why bother? You might just as well die. Or we could re-engineer the brain to dispel all possibility of boredom. But, again, why bother? Our self with its dispositions would have been destroyed. Of course, the transhumanists would say this human self is simply inadequate and should be transcended. That is strictly unanswerable except by saying again: why bother? This could not be a benefit either to me or to humans in general. We would all be left behind. Scruton also believes that such an engineered individual would not be worth knowing:

> I suspect that, although degeneracy of the physical kind might be overcome, boredom is programmed in our spiritual condition, boredom with this life. You could perhaps overcome that by constantly renewing the childishness, renewing the sources of surprise. You would make a most disagreeable human being, someone who is always giggling, always amazed, a kind of postmodern individual, but not somebody anybody would like to be involved with.

I am reminded of Eliezer and his friends.

Philosophers, however, are not consistently opposed to life extension. Steve Horrobin at the University of Edinburgh, for example, argues strongly that the liberal conception of personhood involving requirements like con-sciousness, rationality and autonomy is inadequate because it leaves out the requirement of time. Personhood demands forward-looking elements like hoping, wishing, desiring and dreaming. He offered me a simple thought experiment: 'It is 5 pm now. Tell yourself that you shall have no desires or wishes next Tuesday at 5 pm. That is absurd. You will have as many of those things as you do now . . . Moral talk is talk of values derived from a person – the continuation of the ability to look forward to a future, for life extension, is an indivisible good.'

But the most eloquent, poetic and magisterial defence of immortality is Miguel de Unamuno's *Tragic Sense of Life*. Unamuno, who died in 1936, is a giant of twentieth-century Spanish literature and a philosopher of faith. Faith was to be pursued for its own sake, not for the affirmation of any system or institution. And the key element of faith, the ele-ment that most exactly defines what it is to be human, is the desire for immortality. Immortality comes before God.

Unamuno derives this conviction from an argument that is similar to Horrobin's – that the self overwhelmingly desires continuance. This, he derives from the philosopher Spinoza, who wrote, 'Everything, in so far as it is in itself, endeavours to persist in its own being.' This longing never to die is, for Unamuno, 'our actual essence'. And the rage for immortality is love: 'The thirst of eternity is what is called love among men, and whosoever loves another wishes to eternalize him-self in him. Nothing is real that is not eternal.'

Unamuno comes to the opposite conclusion to the human nature deathists. But this is not because his argument is fun-damentally different; rather, he starts the same argument from a different premise. He agrees that there is such a thing as human nature, but, where the deathists say it is defined by death, he says it is defined by the desire to avoid death, and attain immortality. After all, many things die, but only human beings have conceived of any such wild ambition.

Heaven on Earth

The argument about how we would pass the hours of our extended lives has direct parallels with the debates within Christianity about the nature of heaven. As I explained in Chapter Four, ideas of heaven have oscillated between two poles – the anthropocentric and the theocentric. In the former, heaven is a place where we meet old friends and family, where lovers are reunited and where life is an idealised continuation of life on earth. In the latter, heaven involves a complete severance from our earthly lives. We simply contemplate God and all movement, effort as well as all the human contact that we know falls away. God becomes our infinitely fulfilling totality.

The problem of boredom has pushed the various conceptions of medical immortality here on earth in the direction of a Thomist theocentrism, illuminated not by God but technology. So, for example, there is talk of using the technology that will rejuvenate our brains actually to expand them, a parallel motif to the Thomist transformation of the mind in the eternal stasis of paradise. In fact, the whole transhumanist ethos echoes the Thomist idea of the total transformation that awaits us in heaven. The theocentric heaven is intrinsically beyond the reach of our earthbound imaginations – how could we imagine contentment in an eternity of stasis? We can only understand it by becoming, in effect, different kinds of being. Equally, transhumanists offer a future the whole point of which is that it will engross us in ways we cannot know until we have cast off the shackles of the merely human.

We have, in truth, already started to devise ways of casting off the shackles, of taking holidays from ourselves. 'On the internet,' ran the caption on a *New Yorker* cartoon showing a dog tapping away on a computer, 'nobody knows you're a dog.' The dog escapes its canine self on the Internet. In any net interaction we can pretend to be somebody else. Interactivity is now spreading through all media. The ontological transformation involved is seldom noted. Interactivity extends the self and offers alternatives. I, for example, recently started a weblog, thinking it was just another form of writing. It isn't, it is a performance in which the performer is constantly in flux, modifying himself with each response. I have begun to feel that Bryan Appleyard the blogger is not I. Or perhaps the flesh-and-blood I has become the blogger I. My Singularity is, indeed, near; it may already have happened.

The Real World

The Singularity, however, means that nothing useful can be said about the immortal or transhuman future. The artificial intelligence at the heart of the Singularity will make decisions we cannot imagine for reasons we cannot conceive. All we can do for the moment is, like Eliezer Yudkowsky, try to fix the machines so that they don't start killing us the moment they are able to. Other than that, what happens in the transhuman world is up to the transhumans.

The Singularity, however, is far too nebulous a concept to be taken seriously as a guide to the immortal future. Far more credible – if we take the view that the imminent availability of life-extension technology is itself credible – is to try to see what would happen to the world as it is now. One fact at once becomes clear, the problems of life extension are with us already.

They can be seen in the ageing populations of the

developed world – over sixty-fives now account for almost a fifth of the population of Japan, within the EU the number of workers aged between fifty and sixty-four will increase by 25 per cent, those aged between twenty and twenty-nine will decrease by 20 per cent. Pension funds are everywhere in disarray and companies are having to find ways of dealing with the cognitive impairment of older workers. Meanwhile, hospitals and nursing homes are full of the frail elderly, kept alive by advanced medical procedures. The longer they take to die, the longer the young are forced to stay young – relatively poor and drifting from job to job. Career throughput is slowed by the weight of the old in the workforce. Inheritances, meanwhile, are not passed on so rapidly. As a result, there is a new phenomenon of children living at home for much longer. What they are doing, in fact, is taking an advance on their inheritance. In Britain, there are now 6.8 million 'kippers' – a coinage of the financial services group Prudential. It means, 'kids in parents' pockets eroding retirement savings'. There is, in the developed world, a major death shortage. And here are the immortalists seeking to make things worse.

The death shortage is caused by the century-long increase in life expectancies and the accompanying decline in birth rates in the developed world. Recently, this situation has been exacerbated by the failure of life expectancies to do what they were supposed to do in the late twentieth century – plateau. Instead, they have continued to rise. Even without radical new technologies, the UN expects global life expectancies to increase by another ten years by 2050. Large numbers of people will be living to well over a hundred. Grandparents will have living grandparents. Coping with such a demographic revolution is currently beyond the imagination of any policy-maker. The costs of health care are bound to soar; the old will have to work longer and the young will have to work harder to support the old. What, then, if life expectancies are increased in that same period not by a decade but by a century or more?

Say, for example, the tentative de Grey timetable turns out to be accurate and, within a decade, the first major life-extension successes are announced in mice. De Grey himself says, at that point, 'real pandemonium will hit . . . it will activate a war on ageing in a real sense. There really will be a situation in which people will be willing and eager to make sacrifices we normally see only in war time.' The sacrifices will be caused by a diversion of funds into medical research.

I am sceptical about this phase. Successes in mice may not quickly and easily translate into human treatments. Furthermore, any such treatments are likely to be radical and will require many years, probably decades, of testing before they are shown to be safe. The first very old mouse, therefore, may generate furious debate and speculation, but I doubt that it will immediately lead to public demands for higher taxes to fund medical research, though, admittedly, it may well lead to an increase in private sector investment and a good many stock-market killings. But, if de Grey's timetable continues to be accurate for perhaps a further decade then things might start to get interesting.

Humans being what they are, governments will want to find military applications. Can we make a medically immortal soldier with his fear of death genetically deleted? De Grey thinks that, with life extension around the corner, people will start to avoid risk-taking activities – dangerous sports or becoming a soldier, fireman or policeman. He also thinks that this will be a worldwide phenomenon and so, as a result, the world will become generally less belligerent.

This is highly unlikely. As life extension seems to be approaching, two new causes for aggression will arise. The first is inequality. In the context of the impending rather than actual arrival of these technologies, people will fear that they will be available only to the rich. Currently, apart from notable charity initiatives, we scarcely bother to do anything about the catastrophe of malaria in Africa; we are hardly likely, therefore, to do much to ensure that African lives are extended at the same rate as rich Western ones. The world's poor will not quietly accept that not only will they remain poor, they will also continue to be obliged to die.

The second cause is religious dissent. We have, over the past decade, discovered that, contrary to the dreams of secular liberals, religion continues to be a potent force. We can argue about whether the real motivation of 9/11 was political or religious, but it would be completely irrational to deny that it is religion that fires popular support for Islamism. It would be equally irrational to doubt that radical Islamists would have nothing to say about the decision of the Christian West – and, in all likelihood, Jewish Israel – to extend human life indefinitely. The Pope has already expressed concern about transhumanism. New life-extension technologies may be accepted as an aspect of normal medical research or they may not. As much depends on the rhetoric as the practice. It is perfectly conceivable that the world's Catholics may dissent. That other great religious force, American fundamentalism, seems, judging by my meetings with Dave Gobel and Joe Waynick and others, likely to embrace the idea. Maybe.

As the technology becomes imminent and more certain, more exact problems will appear. I am indebted to Charles C. Mann whose excellent article in *The Atlantic Monthly* suggested possible problems. Will the treatment be expensive? At first, almost certainly, so who will pay? Say it costs the same as retroviral treatment for Aids, $15,000 a year, not an improbable amount. Say 80 million elderly Americans demanded this treatment. That would cost $1.2 trillion, the total GDP of the US is around \$13 trillion. If the treatment is to be made available to everybody, the cost would rise to almost a third of GDP, an unimaginable sum, the payment of which would fundamentally change the nature of society. To prevent this, there could be discriminatory laws that denied the treatment to risk takers, smokers, the mentally ill or just people who were already too sick to benefit. The latter would be a category defined by medical judgements that could be manipulated to reduce numbers. Plainly, there would be deeply divisive issues involved.

Suddenly, the technology arrives. What then? Compound interest is a strange and counter-intuitive creature. Over the short term, the gains it produces can seem negligible, over the long term, they are huge. The rate of real return on stock markets is about 5 per cent. Using that figure, £10,000 invested by a twenty-year-old in 2010 would become £27,000 by 2030. But, if a seventy-year-old in 2010 had invested £10,000 when he was fifty, he would have £115,000 to invest. Twenty years later, his fund will be worth £305,000 against the younger person's £27,000. An inequality of assets has become a gross inequality and the influence of the young in the marketplace and in society as a whole would be dramatically diminished.

There is nothing speculative or merely technical about this. If investment growth rates continue at anything like historic levels, then the outcome is inevitable and the conseqences will, again, transform society. Life extension will produce super-rich old people and, comparatively, super-poor young people. This would be more or less permanently embedded in the system because a much more acute death shortage than we have at the moment would mean these sums would not be passed on to the young through inheritance. In addition, there would be fundamental problems for the pension and life insurance industries. These can be resolved, with difficulty. If everybody was rejuvenated and just died through accident, then pensions could be abolished as people could continue to work, though they may have no financial incentive. Life insurance premiums, meanwhile, could be minimal as death would have become much more unlikely.

If people did continue to work, then getting into work in the first place would become more difficult, a further discrimination against the young. Also we could not rely on traditional forms of social cohesion. Marriages would be unlikely to survive these longer time spans and divorce would become the norm. Relationships would be serialised and love relativised. Then there is the issue of children. If people are rejuvenated, then they can continue to have children throughout their lives. The population problem is potentially catastrophic.

Much thought, none of it conclusive, has gone into this. The most common suggestion is that life-extension treatment would have to be conditional on an undertaking – probably enforced by sterilisation – to have no or a very limited number of children. Interestingly, this turns out to be the deal-breaker for many people confronted for the first time by the possibility of life extension, as I discovered with that stallholder in Cambridge market.

A more subtle approach to the solution than this stark choice is proposed by Tom Kirkwood in a short story he appends to his book *Time of Our Lives*:

In a world freed from the necessity of ageing, the making of children had very great significance. Children were still needed to replace those who had died from accidents or suicides, but the accidental death rate was so small that their production had to be strictly controlled. The method was simple and stark. Each individual at birth was genetically screened and assigned the right to share in the making of a certain number of children. The usual number was two, but sometimes a smaller number was awarded to limit the spread of harmful genotypes. Exceptionally, a person might be allowed three children if, for example, the recent toll of accidents had been unusually great. The bonus of the third child was awarded by random selection.

After the last child a capsule was implanted in the person's body. This would kill them, but to soften the brutality of the process, the timing of death was indeterminate. It would happen anything between forty and fifty years after implantation. When it did so, five days before death the patient's vision would go from colour to monochrome – a nice touch – and neurotoxins would painlessly and gently terminate the individual.

All of which presupposes a phenomenal level of government control over the private lives of individuals. Seeing this problem, some immortalists have suggested that fertility control might not be necessary. One somewhat plausible reason is that, as people get richer, they tend to have fewer children, a phenomenon more or less universal throughout the developed world. If they were even richer, perhaps they would have sufficiently few children to prevent a population explosion in a super-long-lived world.

Less plausible reasons involve the acceptance of an enormous increase in the human population. Either this could be sustained by a Kurzweilian exponential growth in our capabilites here on earth, or we can simply start to populate space. The latter is consistent with the ideas of those who, like Frank Tipler, believe the destiny of the cosmos is to become replete with consciousness. For the moment, however, the technological problems are overwhelming. We haven't even begun to establish bases on the moon, almost forty years after the Apollo landings, there has still been no manned flight to Mars and there is no certainty that it is possible other planets could be populated, even if we could reach them. Furthermore, the known difficulties for the human body of life in space have not been solved and there are likely to be many others of which we, as yet, know nothing. But of course all may be solved by the approaching Singularity.

One problem even the Singularity could not crack, however, would be the speed of light. This is pure fantasy, but it is discussed. If we were capable of letting the medically immortal human population expand outwards into the cosmos and allowed it to reproduce at will, then numbers would increase exponentially. This means the outward movement would progressively accelerate until it approached the speed of light. But we cannot accelerate our colonisation process to anywhere near the speed of light and certainly not beyond. We would be crushed to death inside the globe of our technological capability. The one non-fantastic point of this is that it dramatises our ultimate limitations. Long before our outward expansion had reached anything like that speed, we would have run into problems like the distance of the next planet and the speed of travel required. It is hard to see how the colonisation of space would achieve anything other than the deferment of the population crisis brought on by super-longevity. This deferment may be thousands of years, but it would still be a deferment.

The Almost Real World

To return to earth and to assume that life extension is in the near future, what may actually happen? All forecasts are moot, but the safest are those based on what we know about human nature as exemplified in our history and our present condition.

Transhumanists would dispute that, arguing that such an

extrapolation is irrelevant if we acquire the means to change human nature. But even this amounts to a theory of human nature in that it suggests it is in our nature to change things, even our most fundamental dispositions. And it is certainly not clear – it is incoherent – to suggest that humans can know how to change human nature for the better. We are more likely simply to embed our failings and prejudices in the new model. For example, a devout Muslim's idea of human nature would be quite different from that of a liberal secularist. This points to transhumanism's great failing as a practical pro-gramme. It is no more than the narrow vision of Western secularists, a vision that, in other forms, has repeatedly failed to universalise its doctrine.

But, practically, the first question is: what would the treat-ment be like? Unless we have missed some fundamental fact about the human body that means one fix will cover every-thing, whatever needs to be done will be radical and complex.

In Tom Kirkwood's fictional account the procedure is called a 'fraitch'. In the fraitch, stems cells are introduced into the body. These are taken from your embyro before you were born, so they are undamaged and will not be rejected by your immune system. They are designed to find their 'shad-ows', existing stem cells within particular tissues. The new cells induce their targets to self-destruct to be replaced with fresh cells. In the brain, the new cells are programmed to reconstitute all the old connections, thereby preserving the personality and memories. This is, conceptually at least, simple, but it would be expensive, would require careful plan-ning in the retrieval and banking of embryonic stem cells. The treatment itself would be radical, involving, as it does, a process of massive cell replacement that might feel very strange indeed. Brain renewal, in Kirkwood's story, results in a 1 per cent failure rate that does produce a 'slight disconti-nuity' in the patient's experience. But, by e-mail, Kirkwood suggests it would be painless: 'I think I had in mind that a fraitch might take a couple of days. I think it's likely that the subject might be immobilised/tranquillised to suppress potentially disruptive movement.'

There are many other sci-fi scenarios. In Joe Haldeman's novel *The Long Habit of Living*, rejuvenation is accomplished through the Stileman Process, named after a former British New Labour MP. This is an imperfect system in that it cannot stop brain degeneration, only slow it. In the story nobody yet knows what it means to maximum lifespan, but it is thought to be less than one thousand years. Unlike Kirkwood's neat stem-cell intervention, it is a month-long process involving massive and radical treatments to the whole body. But, luckily, the agony involved is later forgotten: 'The first three weeks were sustained agony, beyond imagination, being pulled apart and put back together; the last week was sleep and forgetting.'

So either it will be a gentle takeover by new cells or an agonising and prolonged surgical and medical procedure. Either way, it sounds expensive. Until costs fall radically, as they might, then there will be an enormous problem in making such procedures universally available. De Grey may not be right in suggesting that merely the distant possibility of such technology will inspire people to demand an instant diversion of enormous proportions of national wealth into medical research. But I don't doubt that he is right that there will be vast social upheavals when the treatment becomes imminent.

Kirkwood agrees. In his story, the first breakthrough is made by a small company, Timespan Inc. However, the World Council on Ethics forbids the research. Timespan goes ahead in secret and starts treating some of the richest people in the world. But the technology doesn't work. Gross deformities have been caused and brain rejuvenation has failed. The rich clients are demented and deformed. A violent and global anti-science revolt ensues. This turns into a vast war in which 600 million people die in the first month. Then, slowly, the world recovers. Research continues and the highly controlled technology of medical immortality is made available to the world.

This version is obviously truer to human history than anything dreamed of by the transhumanists. We are inclined to fight and kill when important things are at stake. Moreover, the way the rich get access to the technology – albeit disastrously – points to the profundity of the equality problem. Immortalists argue that just because a technology cannot be made available to everybody cannot be a reason not to pursue that technology. This is, perhaps, fair enough. Nevertheless, it is almost certain that, when immortality is at stake, the social tensions produced by limited availability will be enormous. Imagine if it happened today and we learned that the treatment was being rationed – either by the ability of people to pay vast sums or by some government decree which would, obviously, involve key politicians receiving the treatment. The world would be torn apart.

On the other hand, the philosopher John Harris has argued that people might not be quite so upset. He points out that we already resign ourselves to discrepancies in the lengths of our lives, some die young, some old, but the apparent unfairness doesn't produce that much resentment. They may sustain this attitude when the technology becomes available. But then as Harris says: 'If people think life extension is good and death is an evil, then it would be mean-spirited to deny good things to some people because we can't supply them to all.'

And, as Steven Horrobin points out, a fundamental change in our biological destiny results in a situation 'quite different from anything heretofore encountered in human history'. The gulf between the biologically enhanced and the rest will be unbridgeable: 'If part of the biological advantage that the wealthy buy confers advantages in terms of endogenous capability and potential, and thereby potential for both wealth, knowledge, and skill acquisition at a level which is simply beyond the *physical* capabilities of the non-enhanced then competition in an ordinary sense will no longer be possible.'

Limited availability of the treatment – possibly a temporary but also perhaps a permanent state of affairs – thus becomes a political and social crisis of colossal proportions. Most will be ageing, sickening and dying, a few will be youthful and in perfect health.

'The gap', writes Horrobin, 'would no longer simply be between rich and poor, but would rather become a categorical gulf . . . There would appear parallel populations in a sense which has never yet been encountered.'

At the moment, though there are differences in the lengths of our lives, we are at least theoretically united as a species by our common expectation of a roughly similar life experience – the expectation of a certain limited lifespan with similar prospects of ageing and dying. Immortalising treatment for some would destroy this simple but crucial unifying force. The treated would have become a different species.

This would, I suspect, leave the immortalised with only one option. They would have to separate themselves from the rest of humanity, creating colonies of the rejuvenated heavily defended against the rage and anguish of the untreated. Since they would, in all likelihood, have superior brains and certainly more money than the masses of the dying, defending these colonies might be relatively simple. At present, for example, though many people in the world want to destroy America, they cannot do so because of American technology, wealth and power. Immortalised colonies would be heavily armed and defended Americas. The Declaration of Independence, however, will no longer apply to these places since they will be founded precisely because, in the future, all men will not be created equal.

Universal treatment would solve this problem, of course, but how would that happen in this utterly divided world? One answer is that the colonies would, ultimately, have to capitulate. They might suffer resource problems or the sheer weight of humanity pressed against their walls might overcome their technology. Or they might suffer internal strife arising from their fortress-like seclusion. They would then have to find ways of creating a fully immortalised world.

That procedure would be difficult, but, if it worked, what would life then be like? The population problem suggests it would be subject to extreme, centralised control of reproduction. Penalties for breaches would necessarily be extreme, anything short of death would seem to be an inadequate response. But, for lesser offences, what would be the appropriate sentence?

In the *Journal of Philosophy, Science and Law*, Richard Haigh and Mirko Bagaric speculate about prison sentences in a world of the very long-lived. The key issue is, as they put it, 'the utility of time diminishes as it becomes more abundant'. In other words, a twenty-year prison sentence will be one thing to a man who expects to live to seventy, quite another to a man who expects to live to two hundred or a thousand. Offences previously considered not worth the risk would suddenly become attractive. Haigh and Bagaric think that, to retain proportionality – the link between the seriousness of the crime and the severity of the punishment – sentences would have to be lengthened.

But, stepping away from strict legal logic, does this make sense? The assumption implicit in Haigh and Bagaric's paper is that the severity of a sentence is determined by the proportion of a free life denied to the criminal. Surely, however, another assumption should be included: that the severity of a

sentence is determined by the actual experience of serving
any given period in prison. Wouldn't twenty years appear as
long to a man who expected to live for two hundred years as
it would to a man who expected to live for seventy? The subjective experience of time would remain the same.

Or would it? If I get up in the morning knowing I have
about, say, ten years to live, is my experience of time different
from somebody who rises with the knowledge he has fifty or
a hundred years to live? The differences in the behaviour of
the young and the old in our present society suggests it may
well be. Leaving aside whatever infirmities may have afflicted
the elderly, they do seem to perceive time differently from the
young. It is common wisdom that time seems to speed up
with age, suggesting that subjective duration is compressed by
the imminence of death. Equally, young days seem longer
and the young seem to think themselves immortal, taking
greater risks with their lives and showing little concern for the
future.

The subjective perception of time, therefore, varies with
age, but is it infinitely elastic? The immortalised would seem
to be young for much longer in the sense that they remain
very distant from any possibility of dying. On the other hand,
certain subjective aspects of ageing would still occur. Young
days seem long because they are replete with the excitement
of novelty. Old days seem short because nothing much new
ever happens. The old, as Marcus Aurelius understood, have
seen it all before. Would not, therefore, the youthful immortal feel as experientially old at seventy as we now do?

This, of course, is another version of the boredom argument. Life has only so much to offer and the soul grows tired
of inhabiting the body. In practical terms, it would, I suspect,
be the central problem faced both by individuals and society
in an immortalised world. All novelty exhausted, people
would become old in spirit and society would become a

retirement home full of people in their late twenties sitting in plastic armchairs, staring vacantly at nothing in particular. Old age would have returned, wearing a sinister, young mask.

This would lead to an urgent requirement for yet more technology to re-engineer the brain so that such exhaustion does not occur. This might, of course, lead to the production of individuals who, as Roger Scruton put it, would be 'most disagreeable . . . someone who is always giggling, always amazed'. But, at least, it would have solved the retirement home problem.

In the seventies, Alan Harrington, a convinced immortalist, came up with a rather more convincing solution to the loss of novelty than merely brain rebuilding: 'A state of indefinite living can be programmed through a succession of lives by means of designed sleeps or hibernations to last for years, decades, or centuries.'

When bored, we simply go to sleep for a long enough period to ensure that, when we wake up, the world will seem new again. It may not, of course, we may wake up sitting in the same old plastic chair. But, if everybody indulges in successive hibernations, there should be some vaguely interesting changes.

Meaning

Perhaps the deepest problem of all would be the ultimate refinement of boredom – the loss of meaning. Harrington shrewdly acknowledges this and offers a solution based upon the idea of humans becoming playful gods. 'Having no clock to race and nothing to prove, this divine man will be free to play, with no more fear of meaninglessness than a football or a baseball player, an actor, a lamb or a puppy.'

Through successive re-awakenings from hibernation, we will toy with whatever lives we choose 'becoming doctor, space explorer, artist, athlete, scientist'. Human reality will become a shifting, overlapping series of role plays. There will be many meanings of life and we can choose to move from one to another. There will be no eternal authority of mythology to tell us who or what we are or what we should do. There will, instead, be a series of playfully adopted meanings.

This will leave nothing outside ourselves to honour or worship. This, Harrington accepts, may well continue to be a human need. And so he suggests that immortal man may come to worship the one thing beyond his control – chance. Chance is the only force that can kill the immortal, the one thing, therefore, still available to accept his prayers and offerings.

This is a very cerebral and probably incoherent solution to the idea of transcendent meaning among the immortals. But it does dramatise the curiously hermetic quality of the extended life. The exit – death – is always distant and we would not approach it through the narrative of a life lived from childhood to old age. There would just be this stasis in which it would be increasingly less clear what we were supposed to do.

The problem is that all our stories, myths and meanings are constructed on death, on a knowable, shared progress from the cradle to the grave. Life, said Martin Heidegger, is a being towards death. Death is not a contingent aspect of the human condition; it is an essential, defining aspect. The highest human emotions are predicated on death. If we live forever, not only will our particular loves die, love itself will die of thirst, a thirst for death. Equally, the immortality of art will wither, partly because art is also predicated on death but also because immortality itself will have become a small thing. To claim of a painting or a book that it is immortal will be to claim nothing in a world of immortals. In fact, since we have only our own judgement about such claims, we are more likely to see the greatest works as absurdly transient as they will only ever be judged by us, rather than by succeeding generations.

Furthermore, there is a deep and absolutely unavoidable selfishness involved in the idea of immortality. Billions have lived and died, why should I in particular be immortal? Why should I persist in being? In doing so, I should be standing in the way of better people, new beginnings. The mere fact that one generation stumbles upon the solution to death does not make that generation more special than any other.

We need death and the dead to tell us who we are. '*Media vita in morte sumus*,' (In the midst of life we are in death) wrote Balbulus Notker in the tenth century. Death is not some distant thing, as our medical technology and our denying doctors have tried to tell us, it walks with us every hour of our lives. It talks to us, the dead babble incessantly in our ears, telling us what to do. Without the ranks of the dead, we should be in silent, limitless, open space, without walls or pathways. All societies are constructed on the relations between the living and the dead. If we sever that relationship, can we even imagine a society?

Transhumanism says we do not have to because the transhumans will construct their own, utterly different societies. Harrington's Church of Chance offers the last uncontrollable vestige of our lives as a unifying transcendence. But this is just a way of shrugging our shoulders and saying we must go on with the project because it is what we do.

'A civilisation that denies death', wrote Octavio Paz, 'ends by denying life.'

The Denial

But we shall push on with our attempts to deny death. Environmental catastrophe, world war, some new plague, some cosmic or geophysical event may – will probably – intervene long before our programme of denial is complete. If we make it, however, then the alien world I have attempted to evoke will come into being. Enough people will endure the 'fraitch' to make a new world of unageing, undying, unloving people. It is what, after all, we already strive for in so many ways. It might be fun. Who knows? But not for us, not for humans, a species defined by death, we will be long gone, forgotten and unmourned.

Select Bibliography

Akass, Kim and McCabe, Janet, *Reading Six Feet Under: TV to Die For*. I.B.Tauris, London, 2005

Alexander, Brian, *Rapture: How Biotech Became the New Religion*. Basic Books, New York, 2003

Anthony, Sylvia, *The Discovery of Death in Childhood and After*. Allen Lane, The Penguin Press, London, 1971

Arendt, Hannah, *Between Past and Future*. Penguin, London, 1993

Aries, Philippe, *The Hour of Our Death*. Trans. Helen Weaver. Allen Lane, London, 1981

——, *Western Attitudes Toward Death: from the Middle Ages to the Present*. Marion Boyars, London/New York, 1994

Aurelio, John R., *Returnings: Life-After-Death Experiences, A Christian View*. Continuum, New York, 1995

Bauman, Zygmunt, *Mortality, Immortality and Other Life Strategies*. Polity Press, Cambridge, 1992

Borges, Jorge Luis, *Labyrinths*. Penguin, London, 1970

Bowker, John, *The Meanings of Death*. Cambridge University Press, Cambridge, 1996

Braude, Stephen E., *Immortal Remains: The Evidence for Life After Death*. Rowman & Littlefield, Lanham, 2003

——, *The Limits of Influence: Psychokinesis and the Philosophy of Science*. Routledge & Kegan Paul, New York/London, 1986

Canetti, Elias, *Crowds and Power*. Trans. Carol Stewart, Phoenix Press, London, 2000

Capek, Karel, *The Makropoulos Secret*. International Pocket Library, Boston, 1997

Carey, James R., *Longevity: The Biology and Demography of Life Span*. Princeton University Press, Princeton and Oxford, 2003

Christmas, F. E., *Survival: The Hope of Personal Immortality*. Hodder & Stoughton, London, 1942

Clark, Charlie, *The Babyboomer's Secret to Living Forever: Essay by a Brat from the Largest Generation*. PublishAmerica, Baltimore, 2004

Clark, Stephen R. L., *How to Live Forever: Science Fiction and Philosophy*. Routledge, London, 1995

Dostoyevsky, Fyodor, *The Brothers Karamazov*. Penguin, London, 2003

Drexler, K. Eric, *Engines of Creation: The Coming Era of Nanotechnology*. Anchor Books, New York, 1990

Dunne, John S., *The City of the Gods: A Study in Myth and Mortality*. Sheldon Press, London, 1974

Dyson, A. O., *The Immortality of the Past*. SCM Press Ltd, London, 1974

Eagleton, Terry, *Holy Terror*. Oxford, 2005

Elias, Norbert, *The Loneliness of the Dying*. Continuum, New York/ London, 2001

English, James F., *The Economy of Prestige: Prizes, Awards and the Circulation of Cultural Value*. Harvard University Press, Cambridge, Mass, 2005

Ettinger, Robert C. W., *The Prospect of Immortality*. www.cryonics.org

Feuerbach, Ludwig, *Thoughts on Death and Immortality: from the Papers of a Thinker, along with an Appendix of Theological-Satirical Epigrams, Edited by One of His Friends*. Trans. with introduction and notes by James A. Massey. University of California Press, Berkeley, Los Angeles/London, 1980

Findlay, Stephen, *Immortal Longings*. Victor Gollancz, London, 1961

Fitzgerald, F. Scott, *The Beautiful and the Damned*. Penguin, London, 2004

——, *This Side of Paradise*. Penguin, London, 2000

Flew, Antony, *The Presumption of Atheism: And Other Philosophical Essays on God, Freedom and Immortality*. Elek/Pemberton, London, 1976

Fulton, Robert, ed., *Death & Identity*. John Wiley & Sons, New York/London/Sydney, 1965

Gaskin, John, ed., *The Epicurean Philosophers*. Everyman, London, 1995.

Gorer, Geoffrey, *Death, Grief and Mourning in Contemporary Britain*. The Cresset Press, London, 1965

Gruman, Gerald J., *A History of Ideas about the Prolongation of Life*. Springer, 2003, originally 1966, New York

Haldeman, Joe, *The Long Habit of Living*. New English Library, London, 1990

Hall, Stephen S., *Merchants of Immortality: Chasing the Dream of Human Life Extension*. Houghton Mifflin, Boston/NY, 2003

Halperin, James L., *The First Immortal*. Del Rey, New York, 1998

Harrington, Alan, *The Immortalist: An Approach to the Engineering of Man's Divinity*. Panther, St Albans, 1973

Harris, John, *Clones, Genes and Immortality: Ethics and the Genetics Revolution*. OUP, Oxford, 1998

Hayflick, Leonard, *How and Why We Age*. Ballantine Books, New York, 1994

Hoyle, Trevor, *Mirrorman*. Virgin Worlds, 1999, London

Hume, David, *Four Dissertations and Essays on Suicide and the Immortality of the Soul*. St Augustine's Press, South Bend, Indiana, 1995

Huxley, Aldous, *The Perennial Philosophy*. Fontana, London, 1961

James, William, *Human Immortality: Two Supposed Objections to the Doctrine*. Houghton Mifflin, Boston and New York, 1898

Jung, Carl Gustav, *On Death and Immortality*. Selected and introduced by Jenny Yates. Princeton University Press, Princeton, NJ, 1999

Kempis, Thomas à, *The Imitation of Christ*. Trans. Leo Sherley-Price. Penguin, London, 1952

Kirkwood, Tom, *The End of Age: Why Everything About Ageing is Changing*. Profile, London, 2001

——, *Time of Our Lives: The Science of Human Ageing*. Weidenfeld & Nicolson, London, 1999

Klein, Bruce J., ed., *The Scientific Conquest of Death: Essays on Infinite Lifespans*. Immortality Institute/LibrosEnRed, Buenos Aires, 2004

Kübler-Ross, Elizabeth, *On Life After Death*. Celestial Arts, Berkeley, 1991

Kundera, Milan, *Immortality*. Trans. Peter Kussi. Faber and Faber, London, 1992

Kurzweil, Ray, *The Singularity is Near*. Viking, New York, 2005

——, and Grossman, Terry, *Fantastic Voyage: Live Long Enough to Live For Ever*. Rodale, www.rodalestore.com, 2004

Lewis, C. S., *Miracles: A Preliminary Study by C. S. Lewis*. Fontana, London, 1977

Linden, Stanton J., ed., *The Alchemy Reader: From Hermes Trismegistus to Isaac Newton*. Cambridge University Press, Cambridge, 2003

Lindsey, Hal with Carlson, C. C., *The Late Great Planet Earth*. Lakeland, London, 1974

Lodge, Oliver, *The Survival of Man: A Study in Unrecognised Human Faculty*. Methuen, London, 1909

Loewe, Michael, *Ways to Paradise: The Chinese Quest for Immortality*. George Allen & Unwin, London, 1979

Lovelock, James, *The Revenge of Gaia: Why the Earth is Fighting Back – And How We Can Still Save Humanity*. Penguin, London, 2006

Lovelock, James, *Homage to Gaia: The Life of an Independent Scientist*. Oxford University Press, Oxford, 2001

McDannell, Colleen and Lang, Bernhard, *Heaven: A History*. Yale University Press, New Haven and London, 2001

Menand, Louis, *The Metaphysical Club*. Flamingo, London, 2001

Miller, Paul and Wilsdon, James, *Better Humans? The Politics of Human Enhancement and Life Extension*. Demos, London, 2006

Mitford, Jessica, *The American Way of Death*. Penguin, London, 1965

Montagu, Ashley, *Immortality, Religion and Morals*. Hawthorn Books, New York, 1971

Montaigne, Michel de, *Essays*. Penguin, London, 1958

Moody, Raymond A., *Life After Life: The Investigation of a Phenomena – the Survival of Bodily Death*. Corgi, London, 1976

Nabokov, Vladimir, *Speak, Memory: An Autobiography Revisited*. Penguin, London, 2000

Nagel, Thomas, *Mortal Question*. Cambridge University Press, Cambridge, 1979

Nuland, Sherwin B., *How We Die: Reflections on Life's Final Chapter*. Vintage Books, New York, 1995

Olshansky, S. Jay and Carnes, Bruce A., *The Quest for Immortality: Science at the Frontiers of Aging*. W.W. Norton & Co, New York/London, 2001

Oppenheim, Janet, *The Other World: Spiritualism and Psychical Research in England 1850–1914*. Cambridge University Press, Cambridge, 1988

Pearson, Durk and Shaw, Sandy, *Life Extension: A Practical Scientific Approach*. Warner Books, New York, 1982

Pieper, Josef, *Death and Immortality*. Trans. Richard and Clara Winston. Burns & Oates, London, 1969

Powys, T. E., *Unclay*. Chatto & Windus, London, 1931

Read, Piers Paul, *Hell and Other Destinations: A Novelist's Reflections on this World and the Next*. Darton, Longman and Todd, London, 2006

Rhine, J. B., *The Reach of the Mind*. Penguin, London, 1954

Roach, Mary, *Stiff: The Curious Lives of Human Cadavers*. W.W. Norton & Company, New York, 2004

Rucker, Rudy, *Software*. Penguin, London, 1985

Sheckley, Robert, *Immortality Inc*. Legend, London, 1992

Stevenson, Ian, *The Evidence For Survival From Claimed Memories of Former Incarnations*. M. C. Peto, Tadworth, 1964

Swift, Jonathan, *Gulliver's Travels*. Oxford University Press, Oxford/New York, 1998

Sylvia, Claire with Novak, William, *A Change of Heart: A Memoir*. Warner Books, London, 1998

Tallis, Raymond, *Hippocratic Oaths: Medicine and its Discontents*. Atlantic Books, London, 2004

Tipler, Frank J., *The Physics of Immortality: Modern Cosmology, God and the Resurrection of the Dead*. Macmillan, London, 1994

Tolstoy, Leo, *The Death of Ivan Ilyich*. Trans. Rosemary Edmonds. Penguin, London, 1995

Traherne, Thomas, *Centuries of Meditations*. P. J. & A. E. Dobell, London, 1948

Unamuno, Miguel de, *Tragic Sense of Life*. Trans. J. Crawford Flitch. Dover Publications, New York, 1954

Vulliamy, C. E., *Immortality: Funerary Rites and Customs*. Senate, London, 1997

Walford, Roy, *Beyond the 120 Year Diet: How to Double Your Vital Years*. Four Walls Eight Windows, New York/London, 2000

West, Michael D., *The Immortal Cell: One Scientist's Quest to Solve the Mystery of Human Aging*. Doubleday, New York, 2003

Williams, Bernard, *Problems of the Self: Philosophical Papers 1956–1972*. Cambridge University Press, Cambridge, 1973

Zaleski, Carol, *The Life of the World to Come: Near-Death Experience and Christian Hope*. Oxford University Press, Oxford, 1996

Index